KETOGENIC DIET FOR BEGINNERS 2020:

Quick & Easy Keto Recipes to reset your body, boost your energy and sharpen your focus| 3-weeks keto meal plan weight loss challenge – Lose up to 24 Pounds

By

Dr. Clay Skinner

TABLE OF CONTENT

- Ketogenic Diets 4
  - Introduction 4
  - Ketosis 4
    - Tips on how to put your body into a ketosis state 5
    - How will you know if you are in ketosis? 6
      - ☐ Increased urination 6
      - ☐ Dry mouth 6
      - ☐ Bad breath 6
      - ☐ Reduced hunger and increased energy 6
    - Is being in ketosis safe for everyone? 6
    - Why a ketogenic diet? 7
    - Benefits of ketogenic nutrition and ketosis 8
- Keto Diet: Food to avoid 9
- Keto diet: good food 9
- Dangers of the ketogenic diet 10
  - 1: Fatigue 10
  - 2: Constipation 10
  - 3: Water Loss 10
  - 4: Vitamin and Mineral Deficiency 11
  - 5: Sleep changes 11
  - 6: Changes in the functioning of the bladder and intestines . 11
- Recommended fats and oils for ketogenic diets 12
  - Not recommended 12
- Can I drink alcohol on a ketogenic diet? 12
- Ready to start your ketogenic diet? 13
- Macros in diets 13
  - Occurrence "macros" at a glance 13
    - ☐ Carbohydrates 13
    - ☐ Protein 13

| ☐   Fats 14

Types of fats 14

   1.) Saturated fats.. 14

   2.) Unsaturated fats.. 14

   3.) Polyunsaturated fats 14

Keto tips to success: 15

   Reduce carbohydrate intake...15

   Intermittent fasting 15

   Empty glycogen stores faster through endurance sports........15

   Consume more quality fats... 16

   Coconut oil and MCT oils 16

   Check ketone levels regularly 16

KETOGENIC SNACKS 17

KETOSE DESSERT 18

KETOGENIC DIETS RECIPES 2

   BREAKFAST RECIPES 2

   LUNCH RECIPES... 3

   DINNER RECIPES 2

   MEAT RECIPES 2

   FISH RECIPES 3

   SOUP RECIPES 2

   DESSERT.. 2

3 WEEKS KETO MEAL PLAN 3

   WEEK 1..3

   WEEK 2 2

   WEEK 3 3

Ketogenic Diets

Introduction

The ketogenic diet is a kind of low carb diet and is characterized by the body learning a new way of producing energy through food. By eating many healthy fats and very little carbohydrates, the body enters the state of so-called " ketosis ". In this condition, the body burns fat instead of sugar as fuel for cell energy. Due to the lack of sugar molecules, the liver is forced to convert fatty acids into so-called "ketone bodies". And these ketone bodies are anti-inflammatory and can help you lose weight. A successfully conducted ketogenic diet must fulfill the following criterion: The liver produces ketone bodies as an alternative fuel to glucose. *What brings a ketogenic diet?* - A ketogenic diet always pursues the goal of bringing the body into so-called "ketosis". In this ketosis, many people experience many advantages over the normal "sugar burning".

Ketosis

Ketosis is a metabolic condition that occurs when the body begins to burn fat and converts it into energy instead of glucose. Because of this, body accumulation - called ketones - is used as the main source of energy. Remember - ketosis is the main goal of the ketogenic diet. There are several ways to find out if your body has reached ketosis or if it has excess ketone bodies. The most reliable and recognizable symptoms of ketosis can be detected in the breath, ketone levels in urine and blood. One of the ketone bodies produced and released by your body is acetone. Acetone is released in both urine and breath. This means that you may notice that your breath has a distinctly "metallic" smell, especially when the ketogenic diet is at an early stage. You can measure acetone in your breath using the acetone breath analyzer (one of the popular brands is Ketonix). Don't worry, bad breath won't last forever, and you can easily remove it with gum without added sugar. When ketones are released in the urine, they can be detected using specially designed test strips. These are inexpensive products that can be found in most pharmacies. They are easy to use and provide a precise, convenient way to determine if you have achieved ketosis.

To measure the level of ketones in your bloodstream, you'll need to buy a test kit (also available in most pharmacies). You need to prick your finger and then place a drop of blood on the test strip that measures your ketosis. Although blood level testing is the most accurate way to determine if you're in ketosis, these test kits are more expensive, so you'll probably choose urine strips.

Tips on how to put your body into a ketosis state

There are many ways to start a safe and effective diet, which is a carbohydrate-free diet.

- Reduce your daily net carbohydrate intake to less than 20 grams: Although it's possible that you don't have to be so raw. Eating less than 20 grams of net carbohydrates each day practically guarantees achieving the state of diet ketosis. What does 20 grams of carbohydrates look like? Try our recipes that the ketogenic diet assumes. In addition, we'll show you meal plans that limit carbohydrates to less than 20 grams a day.
- Try Intermittent Fasting: Sticking for 16-18 hours without food can help you get into ketosis faster. This is easy to do by simply skipping breakfast or dinner, which often seems very natural, because the ketogenic diet is an appetite suppressant diet.
- Don't be afraid of fat: Eating a lot of fat is an essential and tasty part of ketogenic food Make sure you find a source of healthy fat at every meal.
- Cook with coconut oil: In addition to being a natural fat that stays stable at high temperatures, coconut oil contains medium chain fatty acids that can increase ketone production, and can also help protect brain health and provide other benefits.
- Exercise if possible: During the transition to ketosis, you may not have enough energy to engage in vigorous

physical activity. However, moving on a brisk walk can make it easier to get into ketosis.

How will you know if you are in ketosis?
Technically, you are in ketosis if your blood ketone is 0.5 mmol / L or higher. However, there is no need to prick your finger to find out if you are in ketosis.

Look out for these physical symptoms that will tell you if you're on the right track:

- Increased urination: Keto is a natural diuretic, so you have to go to the bathroom much more often. Acetoacetate (ketone body) is also excreted in the urine and can lead to an increase in bathroom visits.
- Dry mouth: Increased urination leads to dry mouth and increased thirst. Therefore, make sure you drink a lot of water and supplement your minerals.
- Bad breath: Acetone is a ketone body that is partly excreted in our breath. It may smell sharp - like overripe fruit or nail polish remover. Usually it is temporary, and it takes about a week to pass.
- Reduced hunger and increased energy: Usually, after going through keto flu you will experience a much lower level of hunger and a clean or aroused mental state.

The above symptoms of ketosis will not tell you clearly what your ketone levels are, but they will give you the answer to the question "Am I in ketosis?"

If you experience all these symptoms, you are almost certainly in ketosis. If you experience one or two of these symptoms (such as increased urination or bad breath) you may not be in ketosis yet, but you are definitely on track.

Is being in ketosis safe for everyone?
Staying in ketosis is safe for most people and clearly provides many health benefits, including weight loss, optimal blood sugar

and insulin levels, and improved attention span. However, some people should only use a ketogenic diet under medical supervision, while others are best avoided. Conditions requiring medical supervision and monitoring during ketosis:

- Type 1 diabetes
- Type 2 diabetes mellitus for insulin or oral antidiabetic agents
- High blood pressure for medication
- Liver, heart or kidney disease
- History of gastric bypass surgery
- Pregnancy

Conditions in which ketosis should be avoided:

- Breastfeeding women
- People with rare metabolic disorders that are usually diagnosed in childhood, such as enzyme deficiencies that interfere with the body's ability to produce and use ketones.

Why a ketogenic diet?
If you are a person who:
- has been using a low-fat diet for years
- eats foods marked as "dietary" or "light"
- reduce insulin resistance
- does not see the results of his sacrifices
- experiences the yo-yo effect

Then ketogenic diet is for you.

In addition, if you are a person who is struggling with:
- high cholesterol
- high blood pressure
- celiac disease
- insulin resistance
- polycystic ovary syndrome
- too low energy

Benefits of ketogenic nutrition and ketosis

1. Anti-inflammatory: The ketogenic diet and resulting ketosis, has a strong anti-inflammatory effect. This is likely to reduce the risk of degenerative diseases such as Alzheimer's and cancer.
2. Energy-enhancing: The state of ketosis helps the cells, especially the brain, to produce more mitochondria. These mitochondria are the energy powerhouses of your body, making you alert and focused from morning to night.
3. Fat Burning: The ketogenic diet can help you lose weight fast and healthy. The ketone bodies ensure a longer-term satiety and reduce hunger hormones (such as ghrelin). This means that you no longer get food cravings and are no longer dependent on snacks.
4. Concentration-enhancing: ketone bodies are an ideal source of energy for the brain. Once the body has adapted to ketosis, the brain can gain up to 75% of the energy from ketone bodies. The brain also benefits from the high consumption of healthy fats, as it consists to a large extent of fat and omega-3 fatty acids support the health of the brain.
5. Lowering Blood Sugar: So many testimonials in which people with diabetes report significant improvements in their symptoms. When the ketogenic diet is properly performed, insulin and blood glucose levels stabilize.

Keto Diet: Food to avoid

- Wheat / cereals: pasta, couscous, rye, rice, corn, millet, bread, white flour
- Legumes: All beans, lentils, soybeans
- Fruits / vegetables: bananas, cherries, carrots, papaya, mangoes, pomegranate, grapes, dates
- Processed foods: ketchup, biscuits, pretzels, cakes, chips, waffles, ice cream, chocolate bars
- Sugar: honey, fructose, syrup, agave syrup, lemonade, white / brown sugar

Keto diet: good food

- Meat: Red meat, beef, venison, veal, salami, ham, chicken wings
- Fish /Seafood: salmon, trout, tuna, eel, carp, caviar, mussels, shrimp
- Milk products: butter, cream, yogurt, cheese
- Fruits / vegetables: avocados, blackberries, blueberries, olives, green vegetables
- Nuts / Seeds: Almonds, Macadamia Nuts, Pistachios, Pine and Pumpkin Seeds, Walnuts, Chia Seeds
- Fats: olive oil, palm oil, walnut oil, macadamia oil, cocoa butter, lard

Dangers of the ketogenic diet

Keto diet, like any other diet, has some disadvantages that you must know before you start.

1: Fatigue

It is possible that you lack energy during the first days of the ketogenic diet. You may feel tired and apathetic (so-called ketogenic).

This is not surprising since the body must adapt to this diet composed almost exclusively of lipids and proteins. Your body can take up to 2 weeks to fully absorb fat energy.

Extremely low in carbohydrates, this diet is not suitable for athletes. People who practice explosive sports such as weightlifters report in particular suffering from poor muscle recovery when they consume little carbohydrates. Some people claim to live perfectly with very little glucose, but it is mostly people with a sedentary lifestyle.

The brain always needs a minimum of glucose to function properly. Certainly, the body is able to make glucose from lipids and proteins through gluconeogenesis, but it is a heavy and energy-intensive process.

2: Constipation

The keto diet can cause constipation. Everyone does not suffer, but the risk exists. Fortunately, this is often temporary and can be remedied with proper hydration, magnesium supplements and increased salt intake (1 to 3 g daily).

3: Water Loss

It is true that the ketogenic diet is losing a lot of weight because the body is forced to burn fat to produce energy. But besides fat loss, water loss also plays an important role.

Carbohydrates retain water in the body. Eliminating carbohydrates from your diet will result in water loss. It also means that as soon as you consume high carbohydrate meals again, water retention will resume.

4: Vitamin and Mineral Deficiency

When you are on a ketogenic diet, you are confined to an extremely low carbohydrate diet. Where the rub often is the elimination of fruit, which is one of the best sources of carbohydrates.

A medium sized banana provides 33g of carbohydrates. What quickly exceed 50 g of carbohydrates per day. Avoiding fruits and vegetables can lead to a lack of the essential nutrients you need to stay healthy.

5: Sleep changes

Because hormones adapt to new energy sources, cortisol levels tend to fluctuate. This leads to changes in melatonin production. Because melatonin is a sleep hormone, your sleep quality may be reduced. In addition to maintaining hydration and controlling hypoglycemia, one of the methods to avoid insomnia is to supplement the diet with herbal preparations.

6: Changes in the functioning of the bladder and intestines

One of the side effects that ketogenic diet will bring you in the early stages is how often you use the toilet. This is mainly due to fluctuations in insulin levels. As they fall, the body processes glycogen in the liver. This causes the liver to release salt and more water is released into the urinary tract. When your body releases sodium, it loses important electrolytes.

It is good to get rid of the extra mass of liquid and water. Make sure you are hydrated and replace lost salt. You can do this with the help of electrolyte drinks or by increasing your sodium intake.

The ketogenic diet contains a lot of fat and protein, so it's important to provide carbohydrates with vegetables.

Recommended fats and oils for ketogenic diets

Olive oil (cold pressed), avocado oil, coconut oil, MCT oil, caprylic acid, butter and ghee from grazing, bacon from grazing, free-range egg yolk, grape marrow, sunflower lecithin, cocoa butter, fish oil, cod liver oil, krill oil

Not recommended

Highly processed oils and fats, margarine, sunflower oil, rapeseed oil, peanut oil, animal fats from factory farming

Can I drink alcohol on a ketogenic diet?

The correct answer is - YES. You can drink alcohol on a ketogenic diet, but you must be aware of the carbohydrates you will be consuming. One beer can have 6.6 g net carbohydrates, while the other can even 18.8 g carbohydrates! Most wines have 0-4 g of carbohydrates in one glass. Spirit often has 0 carbohydrates, but you have to be careful whether it is mixed with something. One gin and tonic drink contains 16 g carbohydrates! Vodka with soda and lime has 0 g of carbohydrates. Like tequila, brandy and whiskey.

Avoid everything sweet or sweetened. Ready drinks usually contain carbohydrates.

Ready to start your ketogenic diet?

Sometimes it is difficult to start a new diet on your own. It is recommended to start with just 3 or 4 weeks on a ketogenic diet. Such a period is enough time to see the results and feel the taste of the new diet, without burdening your lifestyle too much.

Macros in diets

Macronutrients are carbohydrates, proteins and fats. In the fitness world one speaks often of "macros". The body uses the nutrients either for energy or as building material for its various components (muscles, fat, organs, skin, bones, cells, hormones, enzymes, DNA, etc.). In addition to water and micronutrients, macronutrients are in part vital for survival and ensure the normal functioning of the body. Macronutrients provide energy, Carbohydrates, Protein and Fat

Occurrence "macros" at a glance

- **Carbohydrates** occur in bread, pasta, potatoes, rice, fruits, etc. They are almost always in the game as soon as something sweet tastes (except sweeteners). Carbohydrates occur in various forms in nature. Most of them are sugar molecules that are strung together in different ways. Other carbohydrate forms are starch and fiber.
- **Protein** is more common in meat, fish, eggs, dairy products, tofu, etc. Protein is the basic building block of the human body. In addition, protein plays a very important role in both muscle building and weight loss. Proteins are long chains of juxtaposed amino acids. There are extremely many proteins that differ mainly because of their chain length. Small proteins are only 50-100 amino

acids long, the largest can be composed of up to 30,000 amino acids.
- **Fats** are found in oils, greasy meats, cheeses, butter, etc. Fats play a major role in the structure of the cell walls, in the formation of many hormones (testosterone, estrogen and others) and are not least an important energy storage. In which foods is much fat included? You can divide the fats into three big groups:

Types of fats

1.) Saturated fats

Saturated fats have long been demonized, which is slowly being revised. Above all, intake of many carbohydrates in combination with saturated fats seems to have negative effects on many health markers. Apart from this case, the effect of saturated fats in the body is controversial.
Occurrence:
- Fatty Meat
- eggs
- Quark
- cheese

2.) Unsaturated fats

Unsaturated fats are regularly associated with beneficial health effects. For example, this type of fat is credited with preventing diseases of the cardiovascular system.

3.) Polyunsaturated fats

The polyunsaturated fats much good is attributed. A number of health effects such as lowering blood pressure, brain development, cardiovascular and bone health and much more are associated with these fats.
Occurrence:

- avocado
- olive oil

Among the unsaturated fats there are the so-called essential fatty acids. These cannot be produced by the body itself and there are deficiencies if they are not sufficiently supplied. There is a distinction between omega-6 fats and omega-3 fats.

Omega-3 sources: greasy fish, flaxseed
Omega-6 sources: sunflower seeds, walnuts, almonds, sesame seeds

Keto tips to success:

Reduce carbohydrate intake: This is the most important step to get into ketosis as fast as possible. In general, you should limit your carbohydrate intake to 20-50 g per day, so that your body starts faster to use fatty acids or ketone body as the main energy source. Eat lots of green leafy vegetables, high quality meats, nuts, eggs, dairy products and berries. Focus on natural foods and change your diet step by step. Your diet should consist of 45-50% fat, 45-50% proteins and <5% carbohydrates - without chronic disease.

Intermittent fasting: There are no or only little eaten over longer periods of the day. This process is repeated weekly. The goal: By skipping meals, the body is tempted to resort more to existing fat reserves and convert them into energy. So, the fat metabolism is trained. Intermittent fasting can therefore be the ideal introduction to ketosis. You can fast once a week for a full day or set up daily, smaller periods of fasting (16, 18 or 20 hours). There will be two moderate meals for eight, six or four hours each. Example: a late breakfast, an early dinner.

Empty glycogen stores faster through endurance sports: When you exercise, your glycogen stores, your stored carbohydrates, are used up. Since you then no longer provide your body with carbohydrates and thus the glycogen stores can no longer be filled, the body is forced to use an alternative source of energy. The liver begins to produce the ketones and you get into the ketosis faster. So, you can either take a longer and less intensive training session, such as a one-hour leisurely walk or try High Intensity Interval Training. HIIT training sessions are "short and sweet" and very effective. Tip: Exercising on an empty stomach can increase the effect so that you get into the ketosis even faster.

Consume more quality fats: At least 60% high-quality fats of animal and vegetable origin should be eaten so that the ketosis is reached faster. Because ketone bodies are produced from fat. Some good sources of fat are avocados, olive oil, butter, coconut oil, pork fat etc. The quality and storage of the food is always important. Only buy oil in dark bottles, keep the bottles tightly closed and make sure they are cold pressed and of organic quality. Most oils are extremely sensitive to light and oxygen and must be stored accordingly and consumed relatively quickly. Rancid oils or oils of inferior quality do not benefit the health but can even harm them.

Coconut oil and MCT oils: Coconut oil contains the so-called medium-chain triglycerides (MCTs). These are absorbed by the body faster and reach the liver, where they are rapidly converted into ketone bodies. Therefore, coconut oil is even used to increase the ketone levels of Alzheimer's patients and patients with other medical conditions.

Check ketone levels regularly: It usually takes 10-30 days for the body to be ketogen-adapted. To check if you're in ketosis, you can regularly measure the concentration of ketones in your blood, urine, or breathe to control your results and further adjust your diet if necessary, to optimize the state of ketosis. There are three types of ketone bodies that can be measured: Acetone in the breath, 3-Hydroxybutanoic acid, similar to a blood glucose test and thirdly acetoacetic acid in urine, with special test strips.

The most important steps again at a glance:

- Avoid carbohydrates as much as possible (max 50 g per day)
- Exercise to empty the glycogen stores
- Consume high quality fats, especially MCT oils such as coconut oil, to stimulate ketone body formation
- Regularly check the ketone levels and adjust diet if necessary, to optimize results

KETOGENIC SNACKS

Here are some examples of ketosis snacks:

- Avocado with lemon
- Spanish tortilla (prepare and enjoy cold ... gives dinner or snacks for 2-3 days)
- Cucumber with olive oil
- Cold cooked white asparagus with olive oil
- Greek yogurt with a small cut strawberry
- Cottage cheese with 3 raspberries
- Keto coffee
- Keto Chai tea
- Tomato with mozzarella and olive oil
- Kale chips
- Brazil nuts, walnuts, almonds, macadamia
- Sunflower seeds or pumpkin seeds
- Roasted and salted almonds
- Chicken wings
- Pancake soup (with frozen remnants of pancakes)
- Pancakes with cream and berries (with frozen remnants of pancakes)
- French toast (with a piece of previously frozen ketogenic cake / bread)
- Ketogenic biscuits
- Dark chocolate
- Cup of chai tea with cream
- Salami or chorizo slices
- ham slices

- Small salad
- antipasti
- Fried mushrooms in butter
- Macadamia nuts, walnuts, hazelnuts
- Hard-boiled eggs
- rinds
- Protein shake
- Artichoke heart with olive oil
- A spoonful of keto Nutella
- Nut butter - peanut, walnut, coconut
- Eggplant hummus on cheese or cucumber slices
- Cheese chips
- Sour cucumbers
- olives
- Pickled sardines
- Berries with full fat cottage cheese, cream quark or cream
- Raw chocolate pieces (but rather bitter)

KETOSE DESSERT

At dessert many think of something sweet. Sweet = sugar? That does not have to be. There are good sweeteners that can replace sugar and many delicious ketosis desserts. *Here are some examples of ketosis snacks:*

- Fresh strawberries with whipped cream and vanilla stevia
- Cream cheese pancakes with whipped cream and blueberries
- French toast from keto bread
- Small piece of 95% or 99% dark chocolate
- Whipped cream mixed with peanut butter and cocoa powder
- Sugar-free jello with whipped cream
- Keto cake with keto Nutella
- cheeseboard
- Keto Mousse au Chocolat
- Quark with strawberries

KETOGENIC DIETS RECIPES

BREAKFAST RECIPES

CRISPY DRY KETO BREAKFAST
- *10 servings*

Ingredients
- 192 g Almond flour
- 2 teaspoons Cinnamon
- 1/2 teaspoon Xanthan gum
- 1/2 teaspoon Baking powder
- 1/4 teaspoon Salt
- 80 g Butter
- 96 g Erythritol
- 1 Egg

Preparation

Total time approx. 45min

Pour almond flour, cinnamon, xanthan gum, baking powder and salt into a bowl, mix thoroughly. Beat the butter with a mixer for 2-3 minutes, add the sweetener and continue whisking until it becomes light and airy. Then, add the egg and stir for another minute. Add the dry mixture in two steps by mixing with a mixer at low speed. Wrap the dough in foil and refrigerate for at least an hour. Preheat oven to 180 ° C. Roll out the dough between two sheets of parchment paper. Remove the top layer of parchment and use a ruler to cut the dough into squares. Transfer parchment paper with dough onto a baking sheet and place in the freezer for 10 minutes. Remove the dough from the freezer and bake for 8-12 minutes until golden brown. Grease the prepared cereal with melted butter and sprinkle with cinnamon. Although, you can do this before baking to get a "crispier" result). Cool for 10 minutes at room temperature, transfer to a wire rack for cooling and let stand for a couple of hours. Store in an airtight container for up to 5 days.

(Macros - Calories 172, Fat 16g, Carb. 4g, Protein 4g)

WAFFLES WITH BLUEBERRY BUTTER
- *3 Servings*

Ingredients
- 75 g Melted butter
- 2 pcs Egg
- Fragrance Vanilla / Biscuit
- 5 g Baking powder
- 20 g Coconut Flour
- 40 g Butter
- 15 g Fresh blueberries

Preparation
Total time approx. 10mins

Mix eggs and melted butter. Then, add the remaining ingredients (except 40 g butter and blueberries) and mix thoroughly with a mixer Set the dough for 5 minutes and turn on your waffle iron. Pour the dough into a heated waffle iron and cook for 4-6 minutes, depending on the power of your waffle iron Mix butter and blueberries with a blender and serve with warm waffles.
(Macros - Calories 575, Fat 56g, Carb. 8g, Protein: 14g)

CHEESE BREAD
- *4 servings*

Ingredients
- 115 g Ground Monterey Cheese
- 4 tbsp. Coconut Flour
- 3 tbsp. Flax Seed Flour
- Egg
- 1 teaspoon Italian seasoning
- 60 g Salami
- 60 g Cheese Provolone
- 30 g Fresh spinach
- 25 g Bell pepper
- 1 teaspoon Olive oil
- 1 Egg yolk

Preparation
Total time approx. 40mins

Preheat the oven to 180 ° C. Combine coconut flour, flaxseed flour and seasoning together in a small bowl. Grate Monterey cheese

in a large bowl and place in the microwave until it is completely melted. Leave the cheese for a minute, then add the egg and mix thoroughly. Add the dry mixture to the cheese and knead the dough. Spread parchment paper, then put cheese dough on it and cover it with another sheet of paper on top, then roll it out with a rolling pin. Put salami and cheese on the dough. Tear the spinach leaves and lay them on top. Add pepper rings and drizzle with one teaspoon of olive oil. Using a knife, cut the dough into strips diagonally. Fold the dough with a pigtail. Beat the egg yolk and apply the mixture on the bread. Bake it for 15-20 minutes until the scythe turns golden brown.
(Macros - Calories 277, Fat 21.7g, Carb. 7.2g, Protein: 16.5g)

FAT BOMBS CHEESECAKE
12 servings
Ingredients
- Parchment paper
- 3 1/2 tablespoons unsalted butter
- 4 tablespoons coconut oil
- 1-cup cream cheese
- 8 drops liquid stevia [optional]
- ½ lemons, for juice and zest
- 1 tablespoon grated coconut (in filaments), unsweetened
- 1-teaspoon coconut oil, for chocolate
- 50 g bitter chocolate (black)

Preparation
Total time approx. 1h 15min
Prepare 12 small silicone molds or line up a 20x20 cm (8x8 ") square parchment paper pan to facilitate demolding. Melt the butter and coconut oil in the microwave in 15 sec intervals. Add cream cheese and mix well. Add the drops of stevia (optional), the juice and zest of lemon and the grated coconut, mix. Spread the mixture in the mold. Melt chocolate and coconut oil in the microwave in 15-second intervals. Spread on the cream cheese

mixture. Refrigerate until solid, about 1 hr. Unmold on a work surface and remove the paper. Cut into squares, to get 12 pieces.
(Macros - calories 140, fat 14g, Net carb 3g, protein1g)

AVOCADOS GARNISHED WITH SHRIMPS

- *2 serving*

Ingredients

- 2 tablespoonsn mayonnaise
- teaspoon ketchup
- 10 drops Tabasco sauce
- 1/2 tablespoon Cognac, or brandy [optional]
- 14 cooked shrimp, small
- 1 pinch salt [optional]
- Pepper to taste [optional]
- 1/2 tablespoon fresh Italian parsley [optional]

Preparation

Total time approx. 15min

In a bowl, combine mayonnaise, ketchup, Tabasco sauce, very little salt and Cognac (optional). Add the shrimp in the bowl and mix everything gently.

Slice the avocados in half lengthwise and remove the core. Remove the peel taking care not to damage the two avocado halves and place on the individual plates. For better stability, you can remove with a knife a cap a few millimeters thick on the domed side of the avocado halves.

Place the seasoned shrimp on the avocado halves. Pepper. Garnish with chopped parsley (optional) and serve.

(Macros - calories 240, fat 9g, Net carb 3g, protein 10g)

KETO BREAD

- *16 portions*

Ingredients

- 3 cups almond powder
- 1/4 cup psyllium husks, ground very finely
- 4 teaspoons baking powder (baking powder)
- 1-teaspoon salt
- 5 tablespoons apple cider vinegar
- 6 Egg whites
- 1 1/2 cup boiling water

Preparation

Total time approx. 1h 50min

Preheat the oven to 175 ° C / 350 ° F. Oil a baking tin or cookie sheet, depending on the chosen method of cooking. In a bowl, mix dry ingredients. Add the egg whites and apple cider vinegar to the dry ingredients and mix for a few seconds with a mixer. Pour the boiling water into the bowl and mix well with the mixer until the mixture thickens. Transfer the dough into the bread pan and place in the center of the oven. Cook for 75-90 min, until the bread is golden brown and cooked well inside. Alternatively, divide the dough into 16 balls to form panini. Transfer to the baking sheet, place in the center of the oven and bake for 60-75 min.

Let the bread cool completely, then slice.

Attention: It is necessary to measure the psyllium husks before grinding them finely to obtain the good texture of the bread. If you are using ground psyllium, weigh it and make sure it is very thin.

(Macros - calories 130, fat 10g, Net carb. 3g, protein 5g)

FAST PAPRIKA OMELETS

- *2 serving*

Ingredients

- red pepper
- 0.5 bunch chives
- 6 eggs
- 6 tablespoons milk

- 80 g grated Gouda
- Salt
- Pepper
- 4 tablespoons olive oil
- 80 g salad mix
- 4 tablespoons of finished balsamic dressing

Preparation

Total time approx. 20min

Clean the pepper, wash and cut into small cubes. Cut chives into small rolls. Whisk eggs, milk, Gouda and 4 tablespoons of chives vigorously in a bowl. Season with salt and pepper. Heat 1 tbsp of olive oil in a small pan, add half of the egg mixture to the pan. Stir eggs for 3-4 minutes over medium heat. Cover each with half Gouda and paprika and cover for 2-3 minutes. Finish cooking. Half-fold the omelet and keep it warm in a hot oven at 100 degrees (circulating air not recommended). Process the remaining ingredients into a second omelet as well. Serve omelets sprinkled with remaining chives. Put an omelet on a plate. Make half of each salad and dressing.

(Macros 724kcal, protein 33g, fat 60g, carb. 12g)

OMELET WITH GOAT'S CHEESE
- *1 serving*

Ingredients
- 30 g goat cream cheese
- tbsp chives fresh
- 1 tablespoon of parsley fresh
- 100 g of egg
- 2.5 ml of WATER 1 tbsp
- 1/8 teaspoon salt
- 1/8 tsp pepper
- 10 ml of coconut oil

Preparation

Total time approx. 15min

Wash and chop the chives and parsley. The eggs with the water, salt and pepper together in a small bowl and whisk with a fork. Heat the coconut oil in a pan and add the egg mass. Reduce the temperature and let the egg slow down.

Spread the goat cheese on one half of the omelet and sprinkle the herbs over it. Fold together and serve warm.
(Macros - Calories 301, Fat 24g, Carb. 4g, Protein 17g)

EGG AVOCADO WRAPPED IN BACON
- *2 servings*

Ingredients
- 330 g avocado
- 50 g egg
- 100 g bacon
- 20 g of coconut oil

Preparation
Total time approx. 15min

Cook the egg hard. Cut the avocado in half and carefully remove the core. Use a spoon to separate the flesh from the skin. If necessary, scrape out a bit more avocado from the core area, so that fits a boiled egg.

Place two strips of bacon horizontally and on top of a large board. Now place five more strips, beginning on the vertical strip of bacon, downwards. Fill the avocado with the egg and close the halves well. Put the stuffed avocado down on the bacon and roll up. Also wrap around with the length of bacon strips and press well.

Heat the coconut oil in a pan and fry the avocado well on all sides. If the bacon coat is crispy all around, it can be served. *(Macros - Calories 516, Fat 47g, Carb.15g, Protein 16g)*

KETOGENIC LEMON COOKIES
- *12 pieces*

Ingredients
- Cookies
- 115 g (pasture) butter (soft)
- 115 g organic cream cheese double cream stage
- 120 g of erythritol with stevia
- egg
- 1/2 tsp vanilla powder
- 1 tbsp lemon juice
- Abrasion of a lemon
- 1/2 teaspoon citrus fiber
- 150 g almond flour

- 1/2 teaspoon baking powder
- Glaze
- 80 g of erythritol with stevia (ground to powdered sugar)
- 2-3 tablespoons of lemon juice

Preparation

Total time approx. 20min

Preheat the oven to 180 ° C. Mix the soft butter, the cream cheese and the sweetness into a fluffy mixture. Add the egg, lemon juice, lemon zest, vanilla and citrus fiber. In a separate bowl, mix the almond flour with the baking powder. Slowly add the flour to the lemon cream cheese mass and stir well until it becomes a uniform mass. Prepare a baking tray with baking paper. Distribute the dough with a spoon evenly on the baking sheet and press it a little flat with your fingers. Leave enough space between cookies as they spread. Bake the cookies in the oven for about 10-13 minutes at 180 ° C until the edges start to turn brown. Take them out of the oven and allow the cookies to cool completely. Make the glaze by mixing the sweetness and the lemon juice together quickly. Distribute the glaze evenly over the cookies and let them solidify. Best kept the cookies in an airtight box.

(Macros - Calories 184kcal, Carb. 1g, Protein 4g, Fat 17g)

EGG CUSTARD

- *2 servings*

Ingredients

- 3 eggs
- 125 ml of milk (or cream)
- tbsp (willow) butter (or ghee)
- 1 pinch of nutmeg
- 1 pinch of salt
- Chives

Preparation

Total time approx. 50min

Whisk the 2 eggs with the milk, salt and nutmeg. Grease 2 cups neatly with the ghee and fill in the egg milk. Close the two cups well with aluminum foil (I still have rubber rings) and place in a

pot, add water and bring to a boil. When the heat is turned back, let it stand for 30-35 minutes.
Pounce on a plate and divide into bite-sized pieces. Serve with beef soup or broth. Finally, sprinkle chives over it.
(Macros - Calories 243kcal, Carb. 3g, Protein 14g, Fat 17g)

AVOCADO EGG SALAD
- *1 serving*

Ingredients
- 1 avocado
- 2 eggs
- 20 ml lemon juice
- 50 g of Dijon mustard

Preparation
Total time approx. 15min
Boil the eggs, chill well and then chop them. Cut the avocado into small cubes.
Mix everything in a bowl, add lemon juice and mustard.
(Macros - Calories 719, Carb. 3g, Protein 22g, Fat 65g)

PALEO ROLLS
- *6 servings*

Ingredients
- 150 g of flaxseed
- 40 g coconut flour (or 50g almond flour)
- Ground 25 g psyllium husks
- teaspoon baking powder
- 1 tsp salt
- 300 ml of very hot water
- 2 eggs

Preparation
Total time approx. 1h 20min
Melt the flaxseed freshly to flour. Mix all ingredients well and let them swell for 10 minutes. Then form 6 rolls and sprinkle sesame seeds or flax seeds over them as desired. Bake at 180 ° C top / bottom heat for 60 minutes.
(Macros - Calories 174, Carb.2g, Protein 11g, Fat 10g)

OATMEAL KETO

- *1 serving*

Ingredients

- 2 tablespoons coconut oil
- 1 egg
- 1 tablespoon coconut flour
- 1 pinch of psyllium
- 4 tablespoons coconut cream
- 1 teaspoon of vanilla
- 1 pinch of cinnamon
- 1 teaspoon of erythritol

Preparation

Total time approx. 10mins

Add all ingredients to a nonstick saucepan. Mix well and place on low heat. Stir constantly until you get the desired texture. Cover fruit, walnuts, chia seeds or whipped cream.

(Macros - Calories 428, Fat 49.3g, Carb. 4.2g, Protein: 9.1g)

POACHED EGG WITH BAKED VEGETABLES

- *Servings 2*

Ingredients

- 150 g white or brown mushrooms
- Green asparagus - 10 pieces
- 120 g pork sausages
- Roman tomato, diced or sliced
- 2 large, boiled poached eggs

Preparation

Total time approx. 25mins

Cut the mushrooms and place them on a baking tray with asparagus. Drizzle with oil. Grill for 4 to 6 minutes to make them brown. Remove the meat from the sausage casing, crush and fry in an oiled pan. Place the baked vegetables on a plate with fresh tomato. Season with salt and pepper. Add sausage and put poached eggs on top of the dish.

(Macros - Fat 25g, Protein 20g, Net carb. 5g, Calories 345)

CLASSIC STUFFED EGGS

- *Servings: 2*

Ingredients

- 12 large eggs
- 1 shallot, finely diced
- 1 tablespoon Dijon mustard
- 1/2 cup mayonnaise
- One lime juice

Preparation

Total time approx. 25mins

Put water in a saucepan, boil hard-boiled eggs for 10 minutes. Boiled eggs, peel and cut in half, choose yolks and place in a large bowl, leave the protein separately. Add the shallots, mustard, mayonnaise, lime juice, salt and pepper to the yolks. Mix until smooth. The mixture formed from yolks, scoop with a spoon and place in proteins. Serve the eggs chilled. To make the proteins aesthetically decorated with a yolk mass, you can use a cone with a cut end to apply.

(Macros - Fat 34g, Protein 19g, Net carb 2g, Calories 400)

DIETETIC PANCAKES WITH MINCED MEAT

- *Servings: 2*

Ingredients

- 1/2 yellow onion, diced
- 500 g ground beef
- 60 g cheddar cheese
- 2 large eggs
- 60 g processed cheese

Preparation

Total time approx. 30mins

Fry the onion and ground beef in an oiled pan for 5 minutes on medium heat. Add cheddar and stir well until it dissolves. In a bowl, mix eggs and melted cheese until a smooth paste forms. Place 1/4 of the dough in a preheated oiled pan. Tilt to cover it evenly and fry for 2 minutes. Then turn over and fry for another 2 minutes. Then fry the next pancakes in the same way. Add the previously prepared beef cheeseburger mixture to the pancakes and roll them up.

Finally, cut in half and serve to the table.
(Macros - Fat 36g, Protein 38g, Net carb. 3.5g, Calories 520)

CHEESE TACCOS
- *Servings: 2*

Ingredients
- 1/2 cup grated mozzarella
- 6 large eggs
- 4 slices of bacon
- 1/2 diced avocado
- 1 Roman tomato, chopped

Preparation
Total time approx. 25mins
Put 1/4 cup mozzarella in a medium hot frying pan. Wait until it dissolves and turns brown. Gently turn over and brown the cake on the other side. Gently thread the fried cake through a wooden spoon leaning against the edges of the bowl. The cake will cool down and take the shape of a taco. Fry the taco until the cheese is exhausted. Fry the bacon crisp, chop it. Beat eggs, season with salt and pepper and fry scrambled eggs. Put pieces of bacon, fried eggs, avocados, tomatoes and a little cheese on top.
(Macros - Fat 43g, Protein 46g, Net carb. 5g, Calories 600)

BACON PANCAKES
- *Servings: 2*

Ingredients
- 120 g cream cheese
- 4 large eggs
- 1/2 teaspoon baking powder
- 6 slices of bacon
- 2 spring onions

Preparation
Total time approx. 20mins
Fry the bacon slices to crunchy, then chop them into pieces. Blend the cheese, baking powder and eggs in a smooth blender. Add bacon, chopped spring onions and mix the mass. Put a regular or grill pan over medium heat, pour in a little butter and fry

pancakes 3-5 minutes or until bubbles appear from the top. Turnover and fry for a while. Serve sprinkled with chives.
(Macros - Fat 32g, Protein 25g, Net carb. 4g, Calories 420)

LUNCH RECIPES

GRILLED CABBAGE SLICES WITH FETA CREAM

- *4 Serving*

Ingredients

- cabbage
- 4 tablespoons olive oil
- Salt
- Pepper
- 1 tbsp liquid honey
- 2 cloves of garlic
- 400 g of feta
- 250 g of quark
- 1 tablespoon herb mix 6 herbs

Preparation

Total time approx. 30min

Remove the outer leaves from the cabbage. Then quarter the cabbage and cut the stalk out of the quarters. Cut quarters into 3-4 columns each. Spread a baking tray with 2 tablespoons of oil and sprinkle with salt and pepper. Place cabbage slices on the plate and drizzle with the remaining oil and honey. Sprinkle cabbage slices with salt and pepper. Bake for about 20 minutes in the preheated oven (electric cooker: 180 ° C). After half of the baking time, turn the cabbage slices carefully once.

Peel garlic and chop finely. Crush the feta roughly with a fork and mix with the quark. Stir in garlic and herbs and season with salt and pepper.

Remove slices from the oven and serve with the feta cream.

(Macros - Calories 491, protein 26g , fat 37g, carb. 16g)

CHICKEN CURRY WITH COCONUT MILK

- *Servings: 4*

Ingredients

- 1/2 white onion, cubed
- 700 g chicken thighs without skin and bones
- 400 ml canned unsweetened coconut milk
- 2 cups green beans
- 1 tablespoon of ground curry

Preparation

Total time approx.

Fry the onion in olive oil until it is vitrified, and then remove it from the pan. Heat the pan to high temperature and fry the chicken 3-5 minutes on both sides. When it's ready, crush it with a fork. Add pre-fried onions, coconut milk, chopped green beans, ground curry, salt and pepper to the minced chicken and simmer for 20 minutes. After this time, the chicken should be soft, and the beans delicately cooked.

(Macros - Fat 16g, Protein 38g, Net carb. 5g, Calories 325)

KETO MCMUFFIN

- *2 servings*

Ingredients

- 4 Egg
- 30 g   Parmesan cheese grated
- 100 g   Cream cheese
- Salt and spices
- 150 g   Minced meat
- 2 pcs   Burger Cheese

Preparation

Total time approx.

Cooking "buns": Separate the two yolks and mix them with a mixer with parmesan, cream cheese and a pinch of salt. Set aside. Beat two proteins to steady peaks. Gently mix the mixture with the yolks and squirrels. If you want your buns to be perfectly round, use a mold. Heat the pan over medium heat, pour ¼ of dough and fry for about 2 minutes on each side.

Form 2 meatballs from minced meat and fry in a pan until cooked (about 4 minutes on each side). Then, put a piece of cheese on top, pour a tablespoon of water into the pan and hold for a minute under the lid. Put the round shape on a cold frying pan, break the egg into it and turn on and turn on the medium heat. When the protein is set from below, mix the yolk, cover and fry until tender. Assemble your McMuffin: bun, cutlet, egg, bun

(Macros - Calories 538, Fat 41g, Carb. 3g, Protein 37g)

MUSHROOM AND PESTO PIZZA

- *2 servings*

Ingredients

- 2 Eggs
- 40 g Mayonnaise
- 60 g Almond flour
- tbsp. Psyllium
- 1 teaspoon Baking powder
- Salt and pepper
- 60 g Champignons
- 1 tbsp. spoons Pesto
- 2 tbsp. Olive oil
- 45 g Sour cream
- 45 g Parmesan Cheese

Preparation

Total time approx. 35min

Mix eggs and mayonnaise with a mixer. Then, add flour, psyllium, baking powder, salt and mix thoroughly. Cover the baking sheet with parchment, put the dough on it and with a spatula form a circle about 1 cm thick. Bake the base for 10 minutes in a preheated 180 ° C oven. Remove from oven and let cool for 3-5 minutes. Combine chopped champignons, pesto, olive oil and sour cream. Put the mixture on the base, sprinkle with Parmesan and send back to the oven for another 5-10 minutes.

(Macros - Calories 1147, Fat 110g, Carb. 7g, Protein 27g)

CREAMY RABBIT WITH MUSTARD

- *8 servings*

Ingredients

- 1 rabbit, cut into 6-8 pieces
- 2 tablespoons olive oil
- 1 pinch salt [optional]
- Pepper to taste [optional]
- Onions, finely chopped
- 2 pods garlic, finely chopped
- 1/2 cup White wine
- 1 cup chicken broth
- 2 bay leaves
- 1/4 cup whipping cream 35%

- tablespoons whole grain mustard

Preparation

Total time approx. 4h 25min

Preheat the oven to 175 ° C / 350 ° F. In a casserole, brown the rabbit in oil over medium-high heat. Salt and pepper. Reserve the rabbit on a plate. Add onion and garlic and back until softened, about 3 minutes. Add the wine and scrape the bottom thoroughly. Put the rabbit back in the casserole. Add broth and bring to a boil. Add the bay leaf. Mix well.

Cover and bake for 2 hours, until meat is easily flaked with a fork. Meanwhile, in a small bowl, mix the cream and mustard. Remove the oven from the oven. Remove the rabbit, bone it and reserve the flesh. Using a whisk, add the cream mixture to the cooking juices in the casserole. Heat 2-3 min on the stove. Return the rabbit meat to the casserole to warm and serve.

(Macros - calories 270, carb. 3g, fibers1 g2%, sugars1g, Net carb. 2g)

CAULIFLOWER POPCORN

- *4 Serving*

Ingredients

- Parchment paper
- 1/3 cup olive oil
- 1/4 cup wine vinegar
- 1/4 teaspoon paprika
- pinch cayenne pepper, or more, to taste [optional]
- 1/8 teaspoons salt [optional]
- 6 cups cauliflower, cut into bunches of uniform size

Preparation

Total time approx. 20min

Preheat the oven to 230 ° C / 450 ° F. Line parchment paper with a large baking sheet. Pour the oil, vinegar, spices and salt into a large bowl. Mix everything well. Cut the cauliflower into small bouquets of uniform size, then put in the bowl with the

vinaigrette. Stir everything to coat vinaigrette bouquets. Spread these on the plate.
Bake in center of oven until cauliflower is golden and tender but crisp, about 25-30 min. To brew from time to time. Serve hot or at room temperature.
(Macros - calories 90, fat 7g, Net carb. 4g, protein 2g)

CHEESE AND TOMATO PIZZA WITH CAULIFLOWER CRUST

- *2 servings*

Ingredients

- 3 cups cauliflower
- 1 clove garlic, minced
- 2 big caliber eggs
- 1/8 teaspoons salt
- 1/4 cup Mother's tomato sausage
- 4 anchovy fillets
- 2 bocconcini / mozzarella
- Pepper to taste [optional]
- 8 leaves fresh basilic

Preparation

Total time approx. 40min

Preheat oven to 205 ° C / 400 ° F. Line parchment paper with a large baking sheet. Prepare the cauliflower and cut into bouquets and transfer to the cup of a food processor. Operate until cauliflower is finely chopped. Transfer to a large bowl. Add eggs, salt and minced garlic. Mix well and spread the mixture over the pizza crust. Bake in the center of the oven until golden, about 20 minutes. Remove the plate from the oven and add the tomato sauce, anchovies and cheese to the crust. Put back in the oven for 10-15 min. Garnish with basil leaves and serve.
(Macros - Calorie 150, fat 9g, Net carb. 5g, protein 11g)

STUFFED EGGPLANTS

- *4 serving*

Ingredients

- 4 medium sized tomatoes
- branch (s) of sage
- cloves of garlic
- eggplants (approx. 400 g each)
- 75 g of gouda cheese
- tablespoons olive oil
- 500 g of mixed minced meat
- Salt
- Pepper
- 2 tablespoons tomato paste
- 150 ml vegetable broth
- 1 pack (s) Olive mix in herb marinade

Preparation
Total time approx. 60min
Wash, clean, quarter and core the tomatoes. Cut the pulp into small cubes. Wash sage, peel off leaves, chop finely. Peel garlic and chop finely. Wash eggplants and halve lengthwise. Remove the pulp with a spoon, leaving 1 cm edge. Cut the pulp into fine cubes. Rasp cheese.

Heat 2 tablespoons of olive oil. Add the hack and stir fry for about 4 minutes, add the eggplant cubes and fry briefly. Add garlic and sage shortly before the end of cooking, season with salt and pepper. Stir in tomato paste and sauté briefly. Add the diced tomatoes and cover, simmer for about 15 minutes.

Heat 4 tablespoons of olive oil in a pan. Sauté eggplant halves from both sides for 1-2 minutes, then place in a large or 2 small casserole dishes. Distribute minced meat in the halves and sprinkle with cheese. Distribute any hack residues in the baking dish. Pour broth and distribute the olives all around. Cook eggplants in preheated oven (180 ° C top / bottom heat) for about 30 minutes. Remove eggplants from the oven and serve immediately.

(Macros – Calories 610, protein 34g, fat 48g, carb. 9g)

CAULIFLOWER GRATIN WITH HAM
- *4 serving*

Ingredients

- 2 heads of cauliflower (800 g)
- Salt
- 250 g diced ham
- 400 g whipped cream
- Pepper
- Grated nutmeg
- 120 g Gouda Holland young in a row
- 3 stem (s) chervil
- 100 g Shaved almonds

Preparation

Total time approx. 45min

Clean cauliflower, wash and cut out the stalk. Preheat cauliflower one after another in plenty of salted water for 10-12 minutes. In a frying pan without fat, leave the diced cucumbers crispy for about 5 minutes. Add the cream, bring to the boil and remove from heat. Season with salt, pepper and nutmeg. Put cauliflower in a sieve and drain. Grate cheese finely. Place the cauliflower in a small ovenproof dish. Spread the ham cream over it and sprinkle with cheese. Bake in the preheated oven (electric cooker: 200 ° C / circulating air: 175 ° C / gas: see manufacturer) for approx. 20 minutes. Meanwhile wash the chervil, shake dry and pluck the leaves from the stems. Roast almonds in a pan without fat for about 4 minutes until golden brown. Remove the cauliflower from the oven. Garnish with almonds and chervil.

(Macros - 770kcal, protein 33g, fat 66g, carbohydrates 11g)

KAWARMA - GOULASH

- *4 servings*

Ingredients

- 500 g beef fillet
- 5 onions
- 2 tomatoes
- 100 g mushrooms
- red pepper
- 1 green pepper
- 4 pod (s) of chili
- tbsp oil
- 1 teaspoon paprika powder
- 300 ml of water
- Salt
- Pepper
- eggs
- 0.5 bunch of smooth parsley

Preparation

Total time approx. 80min

Wash the meat, pat dry and cut into 3 x 3 cm pieces. Peel and dice the onions. Wash tomatoes and also dice. Clean and slice mushrooms. Wash the peppers and chili, core them and dice them.

Heat the oil in a roasting pan and fry the meat cubes all around. Then add onions, mushrooms and peppers in the pot. After 5 minutes, add the paprika, tomatoes and water and simmer for 50 minutes.

Then season with pepper and salt and open one egg at a time, make a small bowl with the wooden spoon and add the egg. Do the same with the rest of the eggs. Put the lid on the pan and simmer for 8 minutes.

Meanwhile, wash parsley, shake dry and chop. Garnish the goulash with parsley and serve immediately.

(Macros - 400kcal, protein 36g, fat 23g, carb. 15g)

KETO MINI-BURGER

- *12 servings*

Ingredients

Muffin Buns

- 12 Pieces Keto Muffin Buns
- *Patty's:*
- 400 g ground beef
- 50 ml of coconut oil
- 1/2 teaspoon coriander ground

Covering:

- 200 g of tomato
- 150 g bacon
- 40 g onion
- tablespoon of parsley fresh

- Ground 1/2 teaspoon cumin
- 1/2 tsp cayenne pepper ground
- Salt
- Pepper

- 50 g mayonnaise bought or homemade

Preparation

Total time approx. 50min

Halve the muffin rolls and set aside. Mix the minced meat with the spices and make 12 small patties. Heat the coconut oil in a pan and fry the patties well. In the meantime, peel the onion and cut into rings. Wash and slice the tomato.

Cut the bacon into small pieces and sauté briefly in the pan. Cover each muffin roll with a teaspoon of mayonnaise and top with meat, tomato, onion, parsley and bacon.

(Macros - Calories 142, Fat 13g, Carb. 1g, Protein 11g)

TUNA KETO PIZZA WITH VEGETABLES, ONIONS & BACON

4 Portion

Ingredients

150 g tuna (tin, preserved in oil)	50 g bacon
1 egg	30 g of paprika
30 g cheddar (or another cheese, grated to taste)	30 g onion
	100 g chicory

Preparation

Total time approx. 25min

Drain the tuna, Mix tuna with egg to a smooth mass. Fry the onion, bacon and vegetables in the pan for about 5 minutes. Spread tuna egg mass on a baking sheet

Sprinkle bacon vegetables on the pizza base. Cover with cheese and bake in the open

(Macros - Calories 166, Fat 11g, Carb. 2g, Protein 15g)

KETO BOLOGNESE SAUCE

- *8 servings*

Ingredients

- 10 g of coconut oil
- 100 g breakfast bacon
- 130 g Onion
- 5 g garlic
- 500 g ground beef
- 400 g sausage coarse

- 500 g Passed tomatoes
- 400 g pizza tomato can
- 250 ml vegetable broth
- 1/2 tsp stevia extract
- 4 tablespoons cream double
- 2 tablespoons butter
- 2 pieces of bay leaves
- 1 tablespoon of parsley fresh
- 1 tablespoon of oregano fresh
- 1 tbsp thyme fresh
- 1/2 teaspoon cinnamon ground
- 1/2 teaspoon nutmeg ground
- 1/2 teaspoon salt
- 1/2 tsp pepper

Preparation

Total time approx. 60min

Peel onion and garlic and chop finely. Heat the coconut oil in a pan and sauté the onions and garlic. Cut the bacon into small pieces and sauté briefly. Press the sausage meat out of the peel and put it into the pan together with the minced meat.

Now add the spices, stevia extract, salt and pepper and mix well. Roast about 7-8 minutes. Then stir in the tomato sauce, the pizza tomato and the broth. Simmer with occasional stirring for a further 10 minutes. Remove the bay leaves, stir in the cream double and the butter and season to taste.

(Macros - Calories 410, Fat 30g, Carb. 7g, Protein 26g)

CLOUD BUNS (KETO ROLLS)

- *3 servings*

Ingredients

- 150 g eggs
- 90 g cream cheese

Preparation

Total time approx. 20min

Preheat the oven to 150 ° C. Cover two baking trays with baking paper (or bake one sheet at a time, one at a time). Now separate the eggs and beat the egg whites until stiff.

In a bowl, mix the cream cheese with the yolk and then carefully remove from the egg whites. Spread about 8 large blobs on the plates with a spoon and then bake for 15 minutes in the oven. When the Cloud Buns have turned very brown, take them out of the oven and let them cool. Then take from the baking paper.
(Macros - Calories 143, Fat 12g, Carb.1g, Protein 8g)

BASIL KETO QUICHE
- *8 servings*

Ingredients

Ground:
- 30 g almond flour
- 35 g of flaxseed flour
- 10 g coconut flour
- 5 g of chia seeds
- 2.5 g psyllium husk
- 80 ml of WATER
- 1/3 teaspoon salt

Covering
- 100 g of basil
- 400 g ricotta, 45% fat
- 80 g parmesan rubbed
- 200 g eggs
- 20 g spring onion
- 5 g garlic
- 40 ml lemon juice
- Salt
- Pepper

Preparation

Total time approx. 1h 45min

Mix all ingredients for the dough with a food processor and then wrap in cling film. Refrigerate for 30 minutes.

Peel the garlic and chop into fine slithers. Wash the spring onion and cut into fine rings. Remove the leaves from the basil and mince them. Now mix all the ingredients together. Season with salt and pepper as desired and set aside.

Grease a quiche and preheat the oven to 180 ° C. Remove the dough from the fridge and roll out on baking paper. Carefully place in the mold and form a border. Add the filling. Bake in the oven for about 30 minutes.
(Macros - Calories 206, Fat 14g, Carb. 4g, Protein 15g)

KADU BOURANEE - PUMPKIN

- *4 serving*

Ingredients
- 1 butternut squash (about 1kg)
- 75 g of ghee
- 5 toes of garlic
- 400 ml of water
- 1 tsp salt
- 50 g of erythritol with stevia
- 1 tbsp ginger (finely chopped)
- tsp cilantro powder
- 1/2 teaspoon black pepper
- 125 g tomato paste
- 1/4 teaspoon cayenne pepper
- 10 leaves of fresh mint
- 300 g of Greek yogurt

Preparation

Total time approx. 1hr 30min

Tomato sauce

Preheat the oven to 200 ° C top / bottom heat. Now add the tomato paste, 150ml of water, 1 clove of garlic clove, pressed into small mini-cubes, 1/2 teaspoon salt, 1/4 teaspoon black pepper and 1 teaspoon coriander powder to a tomato sauce in a baking dish or ovenproof dish. Cover the dish with a lid or tin foil and bake the tomato sauce for 30 minutes in the oven.

Pumpkin

Peel the pumpkin and cut it into about 1-2cm big cubes. Heat the ghee (also take coconut oil) in a large pan with lid or in a large saucepan. Add the pumpkin cubes and fry them until they turn slightly brown. Blend the tomato sauce with 3 minced or minced garlic cloves, 250ml water, 1/2 tsp salt, the Erythritol Stevia mix, the chopped fresh ginger, 1 tsp cilantro and 1/4 tsp black pepper to make an even sauce.

Put the sauce over the pumpkin in the pan or pot, cover with a lid and simmer gently over low heat for about 25 minutes. The pumpkin should be nice and soft then.

If you want, you can at the end still remove the lid and let everything simmer until the sauce is slightly thickened.

Otherwise, it will be more of a nice tomato sauce - as shown on the bid.

Yogurt Sauce

Press 1 garlic clove and mix in a bowl with the Greek yoghurt and a pinch of salt (depending on your taste). Put the pan or pot contents on a plate, add some yoghurt sauce and sprinkle the yoghurt sauce with fresh, minced mint.

(Macros - Calories 453kcal, Carb. 23g, Protein 12g, Fat 28g)

LOW CARB PEA NOODLES

- *serving*

Ingredients

- 55g pea noodles
- Basil pesto:
- 15g fresh basil
- 35g Parmesan
- 5g pine nuts
- 40g olive oil
- Salt and pepper

Preparation

Total time approx. 20min

The pea noodles are boiled for about 4 minutes in hot water with plenty of salt. You simply add the ingredients for the pesto to a blender. It is recommended to first reduce the ingredients without olive oil and then slowly add the olive oil.

Tip: Depending on your taste and needs, you can now add more olive oil,

(Macros - Calories 707, Fat 55.44g, Carbs 23.96g, Proteins 25g)

SAUSAGE SALAD - ANIMAL FRIENDLY

- *4 servings*

Ingredients

- 250 g Lyons
- packet of corn salad
- 4 tablespoons vegan mayo
- 2 tablespoons Soyananda
- 1 tbsp lemon juice
- ½ bunch of chives
- ½ bunch of parsley
- tomatoes
- 1 zucchini
- 1 tbsp oil

- 1 tsp Dijon mustard
- Salt pepper

Preparation

Total time approx. 15min

First wash the zucchini, cut into slices, fry in the oil and season with salt and pepper. Then wash corn salad and tomato, cut into small pieces and spread on a plate. Put the finely chopped zucchini over it. Then dice the Lyons, mix with vegan mayo, Soyananda, mustard, lemon juice, salt and pepper.

Finally, wash the chives and parsley, mince them and spread with the sausage over the salad.

Macros - Calories 611, Carbs 40g, Proteins 7g, fat 40g)

LOW CARB PEANUT BAR

- 26pieces

Ingredients

- 100 g unsalted peanuts (roughly chopped)
- 100 g salted peanuts (roughly chopped)
- 200 g lumpy peanut butter (or peanut with no added sugar)
- 25 g of cocoa butter
- 2 TL Xucker light
- 1 pinch of vanilla powder or vanilla flavor
- 200 g chocolate 85%
- 1 tbsp coconut oil

Preparation

Total time approx. 2h 30min

Peanut Bars:

In a small pot melt the peanut butter. Add the butter, the chopped nuts, Xucker and vanilla and stir well. Now you take a box shape and beat it with cling film - so you get out the bars later again. In this form you give now the peanut butter mass and distribute everything well. Put the mold in the freezer for about two hours. The mass must be cut resistant.

Remove the solid peanut butter compound from the box mold and cut it into small bars with a sharp knife to make a total of about 26 pieces. You have to hurry up, because the peanut butter quickly gets warm again and smears everything.

Chocolate Icing:
The chocolate melts you together with the coconut oil in a water bath. Now you can carefully dip the peanut bars into the chocolate with two forks and place them on a large board covered with aluminum foil or baking paper. Once all the pieces have chocolate, let the bars cool in the fridge and solidify. Serve cold and do not leave too long in the heat.
(Macros - Calories 150, Carb. 3g, Protein 5g, Fat 13g)

KETO MEATBALLS
- *Servings 6*

Ingredients
- 1 pound of chopped chicken
- 1 beaten egg
- 2 green onion branches, finely chopped
- 1 stalk of celery, diced
- 1 tablespoon almond flour or walnuts coconut
- 1 tablespoon mayonnaise
- 1 teaspoon of onion powder
- 1 teaspoon of garlic powder
- 1 teaspoon of pink sea salt
- 1 teaspoon of ground black pepper
- 1 cup of Buffalo sauce (Red hot)

Preparation
Total time approx. 55mins
Preheat the oven to 400F. In a large bowl, combine all ingredients without Buffalo sauce. Mix well. Use your hands to form 'balls'. Place the meatballs on a pan (with parchment paper). Bake for 15 minutes.
Remove the meatballs from the oven. Place in a pan or saucepan over medium-low heat. Coat with buffalo sauce. Continue cooking until the sauce is hot and have fun!
(Macros - Calories 176, Fat 8g, Carb. 2.5g, Protein 23g)

LOW CARB RISOTTO WITH GOAT CREAM CHEESE

- *3 serving*

Ingredients
- 200 g of cauliflower
- 100 g mushrooms
- 65 g cocktail tomatoes
- 1 small shallot
- 35 g of pasture butter
- 100 ml vegetable stock
- 55 g of Parmesan
- 1 pinch of freshly ground pepper
- 65 g goat cream cheese
- Arugula leaves
- Chives

Preparation

Total time approx. 35mins

Wash the vegetables. Divide the cauliflower into florets. Gradually process the florets in the blender into rice-grain-sized pieces. To do this, always put just a handful of cauliflower in the blender at once. Slice the mushrooms, quarter the tomatoes. Peel the shallot and finely chop it.

Omit half of the butter in a pan, lightly brown the shallot in it and add the cauliflower rice. Braise for 2 minutes.

Pour the vegetable stock and cook the cauliflower in it for about 5-8 minutes until the water is completely evaporated. Rub the parmesan and stir in the risotto. Season well with salt and pepper. Fry the mushrooms in the remaining butter. Arrange the risotto with fried mushrooms and tomatoes and refine with the goat's cheese. Wash the chives and rucola leaves, shake dry, cut the chives into small rolls. Then decorate the risotto with it.

(Macros - Calorie 640, carb.12g, protein 32g, fat 52g)

PIZZA MARGHERITA
- *1 pizza*

Ingredients
- 250 g Bread Fit Baking Mix
- 30 ml of olive oil
- 310 ml of water
- 100 ml of passed tomatoes
- 250 g mozzarella (2 large balls)

- 50 g Serrano ham
- 30 g of rocket (about 1 handful)
- 80 g cocktail tomatoes (about 4 pieces)
- 2 tablespoons of Parmesan (coarsely grated)
- Mediterranean herbs and spices

Preparation

Total time approx. 15mins

Preheat the oven to 200 ° C top and bottom heat. Prepare the baking mixture with the olive oil and the water according to the package instructions and then roll out the dough between two baking papers approx. 3 mm thin. You can make your pizza either round, as in the photo, or as a square tin pizza. Roll the outer edge of the dough inward for a nice edge.

Then season the tomato sauce with oregano, thyme and, if necessary, some olive oil and spread on the pastry tray. Then put the sliced mozzarella over it and bake the pizza for 20 minutes in the oven. The Margherita version is complete, and you can enjoy it as soon as it comes out of the oven.

(Macros - Calories 165, fat 10g, net carb 2g, protein 4g)

PASTA WITH TUNA, EGGS AND CHEESE

- *Servings: 2*

Ingredients

- 1/2 medium, red onion, cubed
- 230 g canned tuna
- 4 tablespoons of mayonnaise
- 2 large eggs
- 60 g grated mozzarella cheese

Preparation

Total time approx. 20mins

Fry the onion in a well-oiled frying pan over medium heat for about 5 minutes or until tender. Add tuna and other ingredients to the pan, then season with salt and pepper to taste. Stir until the egg is cooked and the mozzarella melts slightly. After this time, the dish will be ready and can be served.

(Macros - Fat 37g, Protein 31g, Net carb.4g, Calories 482)

SHRIMP SKEWERS WITH AVOCADO SAUCE

- *Servings: 2*

Ingredients

- 450 g large peeled shrimps
- medium avocado
- tablespoons of mayonnaise
- 1 lime
- 2 cups Friese lettuce or baby spinach

Preparation

Total time approx. 20mins

If necessary, thaw the prawns, then thread them on bamboo sticks. Fry or grill on each side for about 3 minutes or until golden brown. Mix avocado, mayonnaise, lime juice, salt and pepper in a blender. Serve shrimps on lettuce Friese or baby spinach and sprinkle with avocado and lime sauce.

Tip: Wet bamboo sticks before threading the shrimp to prevent ignition.

(Macros - Fat 33g, Protein 38g, Net carb. 3g, Calories 440)

MEDITERRANEAN STYLE MUTTON BURGERS

- *Servings: 2*

Preparation

- 350 g mutton
- teaspoon dried rosemary
- 100 g goat cheese
- 350 g spinach
- 1/4 cup cream

Preparation

Total time approx. 20mins

Season the mutton with salt, pepper and dried rosemary. Form two flat burger cutlets and grill or fry in a pan until the meat is thoroughly fried. Stew the spinach in an oiled pan until it softens, then add cream. Mix thoroughly and add salt and pepper to taste. Put a portion of goat cheese on each burger and serve with spinach and cream.

(Macros - Fat 50g, Protein 38g, Net carb. 2, Calories 640)

CHICKEN IN PARMESAN CHEESE
- *Servings: 2*

Ingredients
- 2 chicken breasts, 150-200 g each
- 1 large egg (beaten)
- 1/4 cup grated Parmesan cheese
- About 55 grams of pork skins
- 1/2 cup marinara sauce

Preparation
Total time approx. 40mins
With the help of a food processor, grind pork skins and Parmesan until crumbs are obtained. Wrap the chicken breasts in the egg and then in the low-carbohydrate coating that you just created. Cover the meat thoroughly. Bake coated chicken for 30 minutes. Use an oven heated to 190 ° C. About 5 minutes before removing the chicken from the oven, add marinara sauce to it.
Serve the dish sprinkled with an additional portion of Parmesan cheese and dry spices of your choice.
(Macros - Fat 23g, Protein 52g, Net carb. 2g, Calories 425)

PORK LOIN WITH BONE IN MUSHROOM SAUCE
- *Servings: 2*

Ingredients
- 1/4 white onion, diced
- 450 g white or brown mushrooms
- 2 tablespoons unsalted butter
- 1/2 cup greasy cream
- 2 pork chops on the bone, about 220 g each

Preparation
Total time approx. 35mins
Start by frying onions in a pan. Do not fry it brown - your goal is translucent, vitrified onion, which has a lot of flavor.

Add mushrooms and butter to onions. Keep them in the pan until the mushrooms shrink a little. Then add greasy cream and simmer for 10 minutes - this will thicken the sauce.

Use a second pan to fry the pork chops. Just hold the meat for about 5 to 7 minutes on each side. Serve them with mushroom sauce.

(Macros - Fat 53g, Protein 46g, Net carb. 5g, Calories 790)

CRISPY CHICKEN WINGS

- *Servings: 2*

Ingredients

- 6 chicken wings
- 1/2 cup hot sauce
- 2 tablespoons unsalted butter
- 170 g Coleslaw lettuce mix
- 2 tablespoons of mayonnaise

Preparation

Total time approx. 30mins

Divide the chicken wings into two parts. Season with salt and pepper. Put the wings on a baking sheet lined with baking foil and bake for 16 minutes turning from time to time. Melt the hot sauce and butter in a pan over low heat, then season with salt and pepper.

Put the wings in the pan with the melted sauce. Serve with coleslaw mixed with mayonnaise.

Tip: Cole slaw is best served cold, so prepare it in advance and cool it in the fridge.

(Macros - Fat 56g, Protein 49g, Net carb.3g, Calories 725)

DINNER RECIPES

CHICKEN CAULIFLOWER CASSEROLE WITH PESTO

- 2 serving

Ingredients

- 244 g chicken thighs without skin
- 112 grams of cheddar
- 120 g cream high fat content
- 140 g of cauliflower
- 45 g leek
- 56 g of tomato
- 28 g unsalted butter
- 16 grams of keto pesto
- 1 tsp salt
- 1/2 teaspoon pepper

Preparation

Total time approx. 75min

Preheat the oven to 180 ° C. Heat the butter in a non-stick pan. Cut the chicken into pieces. Cook the chicken in the pan for about 6-8 minutes until golden brown. Add salt and pepper to the chicken. Mix pesto and cream. Put the chicken in a casserole dish and add the pesto cream to the cream. Chop cauliflower, tomato and leek into pieces. Put the pieces of vegetables in the casserole dish. Cut the cheese into small pieces and sprinkle on top. Bake the casserole for 25-30 minutes.

(Macros - Calories 724, Fat 56g, Carb. 6g, Protein 43g)

PORK FRIED RICE

- *1 serving*

Ingredients

- 1/2 pcs. Cauliflower Cabbage
- 2 pcs Egg
- 2 Garlic cloves
- 100 g Pork belly
- 2 pcs Green mini peppers
- 2 pcs Chives
- 1 tbsp. Soy sauce
- 1 teaspoon Black sesame seeds
- 1 teaspoon Pickled ginger

Preparation

Total time approx. 20mins

Cut cauliflower into inflorescences. Put in a food processor and pulsate until it becomes like rice. Heat a little oil in a pan, add cauliflower and fry over medium heat for about 5 minutes. Put out of the pan and set aside. Beat eggs lightly and cook a thin omelet. Put out of the pan and set aside

Add the garlic to the pan and, as soon as it is fragrant, add the pork belly. While it is cooking, cut the omelet into small cubes. Once the pork belly has been cooked, add pepper, half the green onion and fry for another minute. Then add the cauliflower and omelet. Add to soy sauce, mix thoroughly for a minute and put on a plate. Garnish with sesame seeds and ginger.

(Macros - Calories 399, Fat: 3g, Carb. 12g, Protein 16g)

TOFU WITH SESAME AND EGGPLANT

- *4 servings*

Ingredients

- 450 g Tofu
- 200 ml Finely chopped cilantro
- 3 tbsp. Vinegar
- 4 tbsp. Sesame oil
- 1 teaspoon Finely chopped garlic
- 1 teaspoon Ground Chili
- 1 pc Eggplant
- 1 tbsp. Olive oil
- Salt and pepper
- 25 g Sesame
- 25 g Soy sauce

Preparation

Total time approx. 30mins

Preheat oven to 95 ° C. Free tofu from packaging and wrap with a paper towel. Place under the press, let it lie down for some time so that excess fluid comes out. In a bowl, combine ¼ cup cilantro, vinegar, sesame oil, chopped garlic and chili.

Peel and julienne the eggplant. You can do this manually or use a special shredder to get even pieces of "noodle". Mix eggplant with marinade.

Add a tablespoon of olive oil to a skillet and heat it over medium heat. Add the eggplant there and cook, stirring, until it softens. Eggplant absorbs liquid, so if it starts to stick to the pan, add a little sesame or olive oil. Turn off the oven. Stir the remaining cilantro with the eggplant and place the noodles in the oven, covering the plate with a lid or foil. Rinse the pan and set it to heat again. Expand the tofu and cut into 8 slices. Sprinkle sesame seeds on a plate and brew tofu in them.

Heat 2 tablespoons of sesame oil in a pan and fry tofu in them for 5 minutes on each side. Add ¼ cup soy sauce to the pan and cook the tofu until the slices turn brown and cover with caramelized soy sauce. Remove the noodles from the oven and lay the tofu on top of it. Serve and enjoy.

(Macros - Calories 293, Fat 24.5g, Carb.12.2g, Protein 11.2g)

SPAGHETTI WITH CHICKEN AND PESTO

- *2 servings*

Ingredients

- 2 Medium Chicken Breast
- 2 Medium Zucchini
- 10 pcs Cherry tomatoes
- 2 tbsp. Olive oil
- 2pcs Sprig of Fresh Basil
- Salt and pepper
- 25 ml Olive oil
- 25 g Parmesan Cheese
- 25 g Walnuts
- ½ Lemon (juice)
- 1 Clove of garlic
- 100 g Basil

Preparation

Total time approx. 20min

Preheat the oven to 200 C. Put the chicken on a baking sheet, pour olive oil (half a tablespoon on the breast), salt, pepper and bake for 15 minutes. Remove the pan from the oven, put the cherry tomatoes next to the breasts, grease the chicken with olive oil and bake another 10-15 minutes until golden brown. Meanwhile, make pesto: Mix Parmesan cheese, walnuts, lemon juice, a clove of garlic and 100 g of basil in a blender. Then, carefully pour in the olive oil and mix the sauce. Make zucchini spaghetti. To do this, you can use any suitable shredder or just a knife. Fry spaghetti with one tablespoon of olive oil for about three minutes until the zucchini softens, then put on a plate on

two plates and season with pesto sauce. Add chopped chicken and baked tomatoes, garnish with a sprig of basil.
(Macros - Calories 892, Fat 61.8g, Carb.14.8g, Protein 70.7g)

BRUSSELS SPROUTS BRAISED WITH BACON
- 4 serving

Ingredients
- 2 slices bacon, chopped
- 2 tablespoons olive oil
- 14 Brussels sprouts, cut in half or in four
- 1 cup chicken broth
- 2 teaspoons whole grain mustard
- 1 pinch salt [optional]
- Pepper to taste [optional]

Preparation
Total time approx. 30min
Chop the bacon and place in a non-stick pan. Fry until crisp, then set aside on a sheet of paper.
Add the oil and heat over medium heat. Add cabbages and cook for 2 minutes stirring. Add broth and mustard, cover, and simmer until cabbage is tender, about 7 min. Discover, and continue to simmer, until the liquid is evaporated, about 7 min. Put the bacon back in the skillet. Cook 1 min stirring. Salt and pepper. To serve.
(Macros - calories100, lipids6 g, sugars 2g, Net carb. 5g, protein 4g)

LETTUCE WRAP WITH CHICKEN AND AVOCADO
- 2 serving

Ingredients
- 4 tablespoons sour cream / sour cream
- 1 teaspoon lemon, squeezed in juice
- 1 pinch Cayenne pepper
- ¼ Boston lettuce

Preparation
Total time approx. 15min

In a small bowl, combine the sour cream, lemon juice and cayenne.

Put the lettuce leaves on a work surface. Divide the chicken, avocado and the cream mixture into the leaves. Roll the wrap and serve.

(Macros - calories 280, fat 16g, Net carb. 3g)

CAULIFLOWER TALER WITH HERB QUARK

- 2 serving

Ingredients

- 400 g of cauliflower
- 150 g of Parmesan
- 2 eggs
- 1 pinch of pepper
- 1 pinch of salt
- 1 pinch of nutmeg
- 400 g of quark
- 100 ml of milk
- 15 g of chives
- 15 g of parsley
- 15 g of watercress
- 15 g of dill
- Pinch (s) of herbal salt

Preparation

Total time approx. 35min

Preheat oven to 200 ° C top and bottom heat. Wash the cauliflower and finely grate. Alternatively, in a blender, but do not purée. Rub the parmesan roughly. Mix cauliflower, Parmesan cheese, eggs and spices (pepper, salt, nutmeg) well in a large bowl.

Make 6 taller pieces from the cauliflower mass. Lay the baking tray with baking paper and place the taller on it. Bake in the oven for 20-25 minutes until golden brown.

Wash herbs and chop them small. Mix in a bowl with cottage cheese and milk and season with herb salt and pepper.

(Macros - 596kcal, protein 64g, fat 29g, carb. 15g)

PORK CHOPS WITH FRIED EGG AND BACON

- *2 servings*

Ingredients

- 4 sprigs of coriander
- 1 chili, small
- 2 tbsp organic extra virgin olive oil
- 1 teaspoon curry powder, organic curry Indian style
- 1 red onion
- 1 garlic bulb
- tbsp neutral oil
- 2 pork chops 200 g
- 30 g butter
- branch of thyme
- Salt
- Organic pepper, black
- 100 g bacon slices
- 2 egg

Preparation

Total time approx. 30min

Wash coriander and chili and finely chop. Mix olive oil with chili, cilantro and curry powder. Cut the red onion into rings and halve the peeled garlic bulb.

Heat grill pan with neutral oil. Fry the pork chops on each side for about 4 minutes over medium heat. Halfway through the cooking time, add butter, thyme and the garlic bulb and fry. Pour the pork chops with the resulting butter. Season with salt and pepper.

Heat neutral oil in another pan and fry the onion rings, bacon slices and eggs. Also salt and pepper. Arrange the pork chops and pour over the coriander and chili marinade. Place bacon slices, onion rings and fried eggs on top.

(Macros - calories 1,119kcal, carb. 24g, protein 61g, fat 83g)

KETO PORRIDGE

- *4 servings*

Ingredients

- 100 ml of coconut milk
- 50 ml of water
- 3 tablespoons of ground flaxseed
- 2 tablespoons grated coconut
- 2 tablespoons of ground almonds
- tbsp oil

Preparation
Total time approx. 25min
Coconut milk, water and oil in a saucepan and heat. Add the crushed flaxseed, grated coconut and ground almonds. While stirring constantly, simmer for 5-8 minutes until thickened. Put the porridge in a bowl and sprinkle with an optional topping on the porridge.
(Macros - Calories 819kcal, Carb.6.4g, Protein 19.8g, Fat 74.8g)

KETO RIBS

- *4 serving*

Ingredients

- kg of ribs peeling rib of pork
- 360 ml chicken broth
- 45 ml of lime juice
- 1 teaspoon garlic chopped
- 1 tsp salt

- *Sauce:*
- 180 ml mayonnaise
- 45 ml of lime juice
- 40 g shallots
- 10 g of garlic
- 1 handful of parsley
- 1/2 teaspoon salt

Preparation
Total time approx. 2hrs 20min
Preheat the oven, 150 ° circulating air. Place the ribs in a frying pan or a roasting pan. Sprinkle with salt and add stock, lime juice and garlic. Close tightly with a lid or aluminum foil and place in the oven for approx. 2 hours.
Sauce:
Peel shallots and garlic. Place in a tall container and add the remaining ingredients. Puree with a blender and finely add to the ribs.
(Macros - Calories 609, Fat 63g, Carb. 8g, Protein 51g)

KETO ASPARAGUS MUFFINS

- *8 Portions*

Ingredients

- 120 g cream cheese
- 200 g asparagus fresh
- 45 ml of cream
- 400 g eggs
- 20 g of Parmesan
- 60 g mozzarella rubbed
- 1/2 teaspoon salt
- 1/4 tsp pepper

Preparation

Total time approx. 35min

Provide two muffin plates and grease if necessary. (Otherwise bake one after the other). Preheat the oven to 160 ° C. Wash the asparagus, peel and cut into pieces about 1cm long. Mix the cream cheese, eggs, cream, Parmesan cheese, salt and pepper into a dough. Distribute this into the molds and add the asparagus.

Carefully sprinkle the mozzarella cheese over it and bake for about 20 minutes. The muffins fall after cooling something together.

(Macros - Calories 160, Fat 13g, Carb.1g, Protein 10g)

LOW CARB NOODLES WITH PESTO RECIPE

- *4 serving*

Ingredients

- Homemade pesto with basil
- 1 small onion (crushed)
- 1 garlic clove (chopped)
- 2 glasses of fresh basil
- 1/2 glass of pumpkin seeds (roasted)
- 130 ml of olive oil
- teaspoons red wine vinegar
- (alternatively 1 teaspoon citric acid)
- 1 pinch of salt, pepper and possibly a little chili
- The zucchini pasta
- 1 big zucchini
- Salt
- Cherry tomatoes
- Fresh basil for garnish

Preparation

Total time approx. 15min

First prepare the pesto: Add all the ingredients in a blender and puree all the ingredients to a creamy mass. Try it regularly and season it with salt, pepper or other spices. If you want a milder taste, let the onion out.

Now prepare the zucchini noodles, also called Zoodles. To do this, use the spiral cutter shown above to get long thin strips. With some work, you can do it with a regular knife. With a little practice, this also works

The Zoodles do not need to be cooked, you can eat the Zucchini strips raw. Stir in the pesto and garnish with halved cherry tomatoes and fresh basil leaves.

(Macros - Calories 221, Fat 20g, Carb. 11g, Proteins 3g)

FRIED TOFU ON KONJAC PASTA SALAD

- 2 servings

Ingredients

- 200 g wide konjac noodles
- Salt
- 1 lime
- 3 tablespoons of sesame
- 2 tablespoons soy sauce
- 1 tablespoon Mushroom sauce
- 1 tablespoon of toasted sesame oil
- 1 hazelnut- sized piece of Asante resin
- 50 ml vegetable broth
- 125 grams of kimchi
- 100 g oyster mushrooms
- 200 g of firm tofu
- 100 g of green beans
- 50 g Chinese cabbage
- 1 handful of peanuts
- Coconut oil for searing

Preparation
Total time approx. 30min
Rinse Konjac noodles under cold water, drain well. Roast the sesame without oil and mix with the juice of the lime, the soy and mushroom sauce and the vegetable broth.
Finely chop the Asante and fry in a nonstick pan over medium heat in sesame oil and add to the dressing. Cut the Chinese cabbage into thin strips (e.g. with the help of the Nicer Dicer and briefly blanch in boiling salted water
Also cut the kimchi into strips and mix with the vegetables. Arrange both on plates. Roast peanuts without oil in a pan. Fry the tofu and oyster mushrooms with coconut oil in a pan of golden brown and crispy.
Drizzle with a little soy sauce, salt, pepper and add to the pasta salad. Then garnish with peanuts and serve.
(Macros - Calories 364, Carbs 21g, Proteins 15g, fat 23g)

BACON LASAGNA
- *6 servings*

Ingredients
- 400 g bacon
- 30 g of coconut oil
- 500 g ground beef
- 1 pack. Passed tomatoes (500g)
- 1 cup crème fraîche (250g)
- 3 balls mozzarella
- 400 g Gouda (grated)
- 100 ml organic whipped cream at least 30% fat
- 100 g cream cheese

Preparation
Total time approx. 45min
Preheat the oven to 200 ° C (top / bottom heat). Fry the ground beef with the coconut oil in a medium saucepan until well done. Then add the passed tomatoes. Add cream and cream cheese and season to taste. Slice the mozzarella.
Lasagna layers
Put the sauce in a casserole dish. Then place a layer of bacon on top and top with mozzarella. In this order continue to layer:

sauce, bacon mozzarella. Finish with sauce and spread the crème fraîche on it. Finally, add plenty of grated cheese. The casserole is now about 25-30 minutes in the oven.
(Macros - Calories 997, Carb. 6g, Protein 55g, Fat 82g)

GENERAL TAO CHICKEN

- 4 Servings

Ingredients

- 1 teaspoon hoisin sauce
- 1 tablespoon hot sauce
- 1 tablespoon sesame oil
- 2 tablespoons erythritol
- 1/2 teaspoon xanthan gum
- 1 teaspoon ginger, chopped
- cloves minced garlic
- 6-7 chicken thighs, cut into cubes
- 1/2 cup almond flour

Pinch kosher salt and ground black pepper

- 2 eggs
- 1/2 cup heavy cream
- 1 cup crushed pork rind
- 1/4 - 1/2 cup oil
- 3 tablespoons soy sauce
- 3 tablespoons reduced ketchup sugar
- 3 tablespoons rice vinegar

Preparation

Total time approx. 15mins

Cut the chicken into 1-inch cubes. Crushed pork rinds Whisk together the eggs and cream in a bowl Mix some almond flour and a pinch of salt in the second bowl Put the crushed pork rinds in the third bowl. Coat chicken with almond flour, dip into egg / cream mixture, then coat chicken pieces with pork zest. Repeat until all the chicken is cooked.

Heat 1/4 cup of oil in a wok or large skillet over medium heat. Once hot, cook the chicken in the oil. Whisk together the rest of the ingredients in a small bowl. Heat a wok or a skillet over medium heat and add the sauce to the plan. Once the sauce begins to bubble, add it to the pan and roll up the chicken *(Macros- Calories 481, Fat 37g, Carb.6g, Proteins 31g)*

SPICY WINGS WITH CREAM SAUCE

- *Servings 6*

Ingredients

- 2 pounds chicken wings
- 2 tablespoons avocado oil
- 1 tablespoon chili powder

Optional dipping sauce:

- 4 tablespoons mayonnaise
- 2 tablespoons sour cream
- 1 tablespoon whipped cream
- 3 tablespoons grated Parmesan cheese
- ½ teaspoon mustard powder
- ½ teaspoon paprika
- ½ spoon red pepper flakes
- ¼ teaspoon thyme
- 1 teaspoon sea salt

- 1 tablespoon lemon juice tea
- Pinch stevia
- Garlic powder, to taste
- Salt sea and pepper to taste

Preparation

Total time approx. 55mins

Preheat grill on medium heat. In a large bowl, combine chicken wings, avocado oil and seasonings, then mix until smooth.

Place on the grill and cook over medium heat for 40 minutes, turning every 7 to 10 minutes. (For baking) Preheat the oven to 375 degrees Fahrenheit, cover a baking tray with foil, spray with cooking spray. Put aside. In a large bowl, combine chicken wings, avocado oil and seasonings. Mix until smooth seasoning. Align the wings on the cooktop, making sure the pieces do not overlap. Bake in preheated oven for 1 hour or until cooking is complete and the internal temperature is 160 degrees Fahrenheit.

Meanwhile, while the wings are cooking, make a dip. In a bowl combine mayo, sour cream, heavy cream, parmesan, lemon juice, garlic powder, salt, pepper and stevia. Stir until everything is well mixed and allow to cool in the refrigerator until ready to serve. Once the wings are cooked, set aside and let cool for 5 to 10 minutes. Once cooled, serve the wings with the sauce and enjoy them.
(Macros - Calories 481, fat 40g, Carb.1g, Proteins 30g)

FRIED KETO CAULIFLOWER RICE
- *Servings: 2*

Ingredients
- 500 g chicken thigh, diced
- 300 g cauliflower rubella
- 2 tablespoons of butter
- 50 g grated carrots
- 50 g chopped broccoli

Preparation
Total time approx. 25mins
Put the chopped chicken in an oiled wok or deep frying pan and fry for five minutes. At the same time, crush the cauliflower so that it resembles rice. Mix the cauliflower with chicken in the pan, add broccoli, butter, carrots and fry for another 5 to 8 minutes, stirring constantly. Salt and pepper well before serving
(Macros - Fat 20g, Protein 52g, Net carb. 5g, Calories420)

SALAD WITH CHICKEN AND AVOCADO
- *Servings: 2*

Ingredients
- 220 g chicken thighs, boneless and skinless
- 1 medium avocado
- 2 Roman tomatoes
- 1 handful of lettuce
- Juice of 1 lime

Preparation
Total time approx. 20mins

Grill or fry the legs until completely soft. About 5-8 minutes on each side. Cut the tomatoes and avocados into cubes or slices. Tear the lettuce into bite-sized pieces. Crumble chicken legs with forks and combine all ingredients in a large bowl. Add whole lime juice. Season with salt and pepper to taste. Mix and enjoy the taste!
(Macros - Fat 16g, Protein 32g, Net carb. 4g, Calories 300)

SPICY NUT MIX

- *2 servings*

Ingredients

- 100 g almonds
- 100 g of cashew nuts
- 75 g walnuts
- 50 g sunflower seeds
- 1 teaspoon smoked paprika powder
- 1 tsp chili flakes
- 1/2 teaspoon fine Himalayan salt
- 1 tsp garlic powder
- 1 tbsp avocado oil

Preparation

Total time approx. 30mins

Preheat the oven to 175 degrees Celsius and lay out a baking tray with baking paper. Mix all the nuts and seeds together and put them in a thin layer on the baking tray. Roast the nuts for 10 - 15 minutes in the oven. You always turn it after 5 minutes. In the meantime mix salt, spices and oil. Let the nuts cool for a few minutes, then put them in a large bowl and add the spice mixture. Mix nuts and spice mixture thoroughly and let cool completely. You can now keep the nuts in an airtight container for a few days.
(Macros - Calorie 2086, fat 46g, net carb. 14.8g, 70g protein)

MEAT RECIPES

RIB EYE STEAK
- *2 servings*

Ingredients
- 2 entrecote steaks
- 2 tablespoons vegetable oil
- Sea-salt
- Freshly ground pepper

Preparation

Total time approx. 20min

Wash meat and pat dry. Heat cast-iron pan or grill pan and add oil. When the oil is hot, sauté meat from both sides for about 2 minutes. Cook in preheated oven at 130 ° C for about 5-10 minutes, the core temperature of the meat should be about 54 ° C. Remove, season with salt and pepper from both sides and let stand covered for approx. 4 minutes.

(Macros - 400kcal, protein 44g, fat 25g, carb. 0g)

TENDER BEEF WITH BROCCOLI
- *Servings: 2*

Ingredients
- 100 g broccoli
- 1 clove of garlic
- About 500 g of ground beef
- 125 g grated mozzarella cheese
- 1 large egg

Preparation

Total time approx. 30mins

Cut the broccoli and sauté the florets on high heat for about 5-8 minutes. Press the garlic through the press or finely sieve and add to the broccoli. Cook garlic and broccoli until tender. Add ground beef to broccoli and garlic and fry for a few minutes until the meat changes its structure. Add grated mozzarella cheese and beat in the egg so that all the ingredients combine well. Add salt and pepper to taste and serve immediately after removing from the pan.

(Macros - Fat 41g, Protein 60g, Net carb. 5g, Calories 660)

BEEF PATCH STEAK WITH ASPARAGUS

- *Servings: 2*

Ingredients

- 16 asparagus
- 350 g beef patch
- 175 g mushrooms or forest mushrooms
- 1 clove of garlic
- 1/4 cup of thick cream (preferably 36%)

Preparation

Total time approx. 30mins

Cut off the fibrous tip with asparagus thickening and bake at 200 ° C for 15 minutes.

Rub the steaks with salt and pepper, then bake on a wire rack or grill pan for 10 minutes - 5 minutes on each side.

Cook mushrooms or forest mushrooms with the addition of garlic squeezed in a well-oiled pan for 8 minutes. After this time, add thick cream, mix well and leave to thicken.

After frying the steaks, cover them with aluminum foil and leave the meat under the foil for about 5 minutes. After this time, cut the beef, pour the cream-mushroom sauce and serve with baked asparagus.

(Macros - Fat 27g, Protein 38g, Net carb. 5g, Calorie 445)

BEEF MEATBALLS WITH PARMESAN CHEESE

- *Servings: 2*

Ingredients

- 500 g ground beef
- 1 egg (beaten)
- 1/4 cup grated Parmesan cheese
- 1/2 cup marinara sauce
- 200 g zucchini

Preparation

Total time approx. 25mins

Mix the beef, beaten egg and Parmesan cheese with the spices of your choice. Create balls with a diameter of about 2.5 cm. Fry the meatballs on each side over high heat. Then reduce it, add marinara sauce and cook covered for 10 minutes.

Make zucchini pasta (preferably use a vegetable spiralizer) and fry it with a small amount of oil for no more than 2 minutes. Remember to constantly stir or toss it in the pan. Add meatballs on top of zucchini pasta.

(Macros - Fat 35g, Protein 52g, Net carb. 4g, Calories 575)

CHICKEN SATAY

- 4 serving

Ingredients

- 400 g chicken breast
- Salt
- 3.5 tbsp oil
- 1 red chili pepper
- 150 ml of coconut milk
- 3 tablespoons of peanut butter
- 1 tbsp light soy sauce

Preparation

Total time approx. 25min

Wash chicken, pat dry and cut into thin strips. Wave the meat on skewers. Season with salt. Heat 2-3 tablespoons of oil in a pan and fry the skewers in 2 portions from each side for about 3 minutes. Slice the chili pepper lengthwise, remove the seeds and chop the chili pepper. Heat 1 tbsp of oil in a small saucepan and sauté the chili. Add coconut milk, peanut butter and soy sauce, stir and bring to a boil. Simmer the sauce for 1-2 minutes and serve with the skewers.

(Macros - 187kcal, protein 26g, fat 8g, carb. 2g)

LOW CARB BEEF FILLET ON ROASTED CAULIFLOWER WITH YOGHURT & POMEGRANATE

- 4 serving

Ingredients

- head cauliflower
- 1 pomegranate
- 500 g of yogurt
- Fresh ginger (2 cm)
- 1 organic orange
- 1 organic lemon
- Salt

Pepper

- 800 g beef fillet
- 3 teaspoons olive oil
- 1 bunch of parsley
- 100 g almond flakes
- 4 teaspoons honey

Preparation
Total time approx. 30min

Clean the cauliflower and remove the florets. Cut the top of the florets off the stem and cut them with your hands. Add the cauliflower to the cold pan, then turn up the heat and roast the cauliflower from all sides while stirring. Separate the stalk from the pomegranate and halve the pomegranate. Dissolve cores. Turn cauliflower over, turn down temperature to medium heat.

Smooth yoghurt in a mixing bowl until smooth. Peel ginger and rub over the yoghurt. Wash hot orange and lemon and finely chop the skin. In each case squeeze the juice of ½ orange and ½ lemon. Mix the peel and juice under the yoghurt. Season with salt and pepper.

Wash beef fillet, pat dry and cut into steaks. Heat cast-iron pan and brush with 1 teaspoon of oil. Fry steaks in the hot pan from both sides for 3-4 minutes. While frying the steaks, add 2 teaspoons of olive oil and the almonds to the cauliflower, stir and roast briefly. Season with salt and pepper. Season meat with salt and pepper. Chop parsley. Put some yoghurt on a plate and add ¼ of cauliflower. Sprinkle with pomegranate seeds. Arrange 1 steak on each and drizzle with 1 teaspoon of honey. Sprinkle with parsley.

(Macros - 536kcal, protein 52g, fat 28g, carb. 15g)

ROAST BEEF
- *6 servings*

Ingredients
- 1.5 kg of roast beef
- 1 tbsp salt
- 2 tbsp black peppercorns
- Oil
- 2 branch (s) of rosemary

Preparation
Total time approx. 90min

Remove the roast beef from the refrigerator about 2 hours before frying and bring to room temperature. Grind the salt and pepper in a mortar and rub the roast beef well from all sides.

Sauté the roast beef on the side with the fat layer in oil for about 3 minutes.

Place the meat on the baking tray with the sides side up, sprinkle with the rosemary needles and place in the preheated oven (95 ° C, top / bottom heat). Cover with oil and fry until the core temperature reaches 58 ° C. That takes about an hour. Then rest for 20 minutes.

(Macros - 371kcal, protein 56g, fat 15g, carb. 0g)

BEEF AND FOREST MUSHROOM

- *4 servings*

Ingredients

- 110 g Butter
- 300 g Forest mushrooms
- 1 White onion
- 2 Bell peppers
- 450 g Beef tenderloin, finely chopped
- 1 Head of garlic
- 1 teaspoon Italian herbs
- 200 g Cheese Provolone
- Salt and pepper
- 4 tbsp. Marinara sauce (tomato) without sugar
- 4 tbsp. Olive oil

Preparation

Total time approx. 30mins

Slice the mushrooms, onions and peppers. Lightly fry in butter for 2-3 minutes and transfer to a bowl. In the same pan, fry the beef for five minutes, add the garlic, salt and pepper. Return the vegetables and fry for another 3-5 minutes, sprinkle with Italian herbs. Put everything in a baking dish, sprinkle with grated cheese and send to the oven preheated to 225 ° C for 15 minutes or until the casserole is covered with a golden crust. Remove from the oven, grease with tomato sauce and lightly pour olive oil

(Macros - Calories 806, Fat 68g, Protein 40g)

CASSEROLE CHICKEN AND BROCCOLI

- *Servings: 4*

Ingredients

- 500 g chicken thigh meat
- 3 cups of broccoli florets
- 1/2 cup mayonnaise
- 2 and 1/2 cups grated cheddar cheese
- 1 fresh green jalapeno pepper – sliced

Preparation

Total time approx. 65mins

Fry chicken meat over medium heat in a well-oiled pan. Separate them with two forks or a special meat chopper. Chop the broccoli and combine it with mayonnaise, 2 glasses of cheddar, season with salt and pepper. Then, transfer to an ovenproof 23x33 cm dish. Bake for 25 minutes at 180 degrees Celsius. Five minutes before the end of baking, the rest of the cheese and the sharpest jalapeno pepper will go to the casserole - sprinkle the top of the dish with them.

(Macros - Fat 47g, Protein 44g, Net carb. 5g, Calorie 610)

CHINESE STYLE BEEF WITH VEGETABLES

- *Servings: 4*

Ingredients

- medium carrot
- 1 small green cabbage
- 500 g ground beef
- 2 tbsp soy sauce
- 1 fresh chives

Preparation

Total time approx. 25mins

Cut the carrots and small cabbage. Put ground beef in a large frying pan or wok, crush into small pieces with a spoon, heat to brown. About 5-10 minutes after browning, add chopped carrots, cabbage, soy sauce. Salt and pepper to taste. Mix the ingredients and simmer for 5 minutes or until the cabbage "withers".
Serve with chopped chives.

(Macros - Fat 26g, Protein 48g, Net Carb 5g, Calorie 480)

LASAGNE WITH MINCED MEAT AND ZUCCHINI

- *Servings: 4*

Ingredients

- 450 g ground beef
- A glass of marinara sauce
- Large zucchini
- 280 g ricotta cheese
- 115 g of crushed mozzarella

Preparation

Total time approx. 70mins

Preheat the oven to 180 degrees Celsius. Cut the zucchini into thin strips, the easiest way to do this is with a vegetable peeler. Then salt them and let stand for 15 minutes. After this time, squeeze out the excess water with clean kitchen paper.

Fry ground beef in an oiled pan. Add marinara sauce and season with pepper and salt.

Arrange the layers in a 9x9 heat resistant dish: minced meat, zucchini strips, ricotta, meat, zucchini strips, ricotta and mozzarella.

Cover the dish with foil and bake for 30 minutes. Finally remove the foil and fry for 2-3 minutes to caramelize the top.

(Macros - Fat 46g, Protein 33g, Net carb.5g, Calories 573)

SWEET PORK TENDERLOIN

- *Servings: 2*

Ingredients

- 750 g of pork
- 40 g chopped apples
- 2-4 sprigs of rosemary
- 4 tablespoons unsalted butter
- 200 g cauliflower

Preparation

Total time approx. 30mins

Season the pork chop with salt and pepper, then fry on both sides on high heat in a well-oiled pan. Reduce heat and add a chopped apple and place a sprig of rosemary on top of the loin. Cover the pan and simmer for about 8 minutes. Steam the cauliflower, mix with butter and season with salt and pepper. The prepared meat

should be served with a fresh sprig of rosemary and cauliflower puree.
(Macros - Fat 28g, Protein 37g, Net carb.5g, Calories 420)

COD COOKED WITH MARINARA SAUCE

- *Servings: 2*

Ingredients

- 2 fillets of cod, approx. 250 g
- 2 teaspoons of olive oil
- 1/2 cup herb-tomato marinara sauce
- 3 bay leaves
- 2 cups green beans

Preparation
Total time approx. 20mins
Heat the olive oil with the marinara sauce over medium heat. Add bay leaves, a pinch of pepper and salt to taste, and then pour a glass of water. The whole choke for about 5 minutes.
Reduce the flame under the pan and add the cod fillets. Cover and simmer for 10 minutes, in the meantime turning over the fillets.
In a second frying pan, sauté the green beans in a tablespoon of olive oil and keep on medium heat for about 10 minutes.
When the cod fillet is stewed and its meat is opaque, the dish is ready. Serve with warm beans.
(Macros - Fat 20g, Protein 43g, Net carb. 5g, Calories 390)

MEATBALLS ON BEETROOT VEGETABLES

- *2 servings*

Ingredients

- Walnut kernels, whole
- 2 tbsp olive oil
- Sea salt
- Pepper
- 4 branch (s) of rosemary
- 400 g minced meat, mixed
- 1 egg
- 2 tsp curry powder
- 2 teaspoons paprika powder
- 2 tbsp neutral oil
- 3 branch(s) of thyme
- 500 g beetroot, pre-cooked
- 1 clove of garlic
- 2 shallots
- 25 g of butter

- 1 tsp caraway
- 1 tbsp red wine vinegar

Preparation

Total time approx. 40min

Hop the walnuts and mix with the olive oil. Salting and peppering. Pluck rosemary needles and chop. Mix the minced meat with the egg, curry powder, paprika and rosemary. Season with sea salt and pepper. From the mince form small balls. Heat neutral oil in a pan and fry the meatballs with the thyme sprigs over medium heat and cook. Then cut the beetroot into slices. Peel and finely chop the garlic and shallots. Heat butter in a saucepan. Heat the cumin, shallots, garlic and beetroot for about 5 minutes over medium heat.

Season with sea salt, pepper and red wine vinegar. Arrange the beetroot vegetables with the meatballs and drizzle with the walnut pesto. If you like, you can garnish it with a sprig of fresh marjoram. (Macros - calories 670, carb. 36g, protein 13g, fat 50g)

TURKEY SLICES WITH ZUCCHINI AND FENNEL

- *4 servings*

Ingredients

- 500 g of turkey meat
- 30 g coconut oil (for searing)
- 1 zucchini (300g)
- 1 fennel tuber
- 100 g crème fraîche
- 100 g cream cheese
- 1 onion
- Salt
- Pepper
- Herbs (at will)

Preparation

Total time approx. 35min

First cut the turkey into small, bite-sized pieces, season with salt and pepper and set aside again. Now cut the onion into small cubes and, together with the coconut oil, sauté in a large pan.

Add the pieces of meat and fry well from all sides. In the meantime, quarter the zucchini and cut into small pieces. With the fennel tuber cut away the root, the upper Strunk as well, but this set aside, we still need. Then quarter the fennel tuber and cut into slices. When the meat is well-fried, add zucchini and fennel. Continue to simmer together for about 10 minutes. Meanwhile, finely chop the upper stem of the fennel with the fine leaves.

If there is no water left in the pan, deglaze everything with a little water. Then add creme fraiche and cream cheese and mix well with meat and vegetables. Strain the sauce with water to the desired consistency. Season to taste with salt, pepper and herbs. Finally, as a decoration to give the fine fennel leaves on the sliced.
(Macros - Calories 379, Carb. 5g, Protein 33g, Fat 23g)

FISH RECIPES

SALMON CUTLETS WITH FRESH HERBS

- *5 servings*

Ingredients

- 500 ml Canned salmon
- 2 tbsp. Chopped Chives
- 50 ml Finely chopped dill
- 25 g Parmesan Cheese
- 120 g Ground Bacon
- 2 Eggs
- 1 teaspoon Lemon zest
- Salt and pepper
- 100 ml Almond flour
- 2 tbsp. Olive oil

Preparation

Total time approx. 30mins

Open the canned food, drain the liquid and transfer to a large bowl. Add onions, dill, parmesan, crushed bacon, two large eggs, lemon zest, salt and pepper, mix everything thoroughly. Divide the minced meat into cutlets weighing about 90 grams. It should turn out 10 pieces. Pour almond flour into a plate, carefully roll cutlets in it (they are fragile). Heat 2 tbsp of olive oil in a pan. Sauté the meatballs on medium heat until golden on each side. Put two meatballs, broccoli in a bowl and season with tartar sauce.

(Macros - Calories 418, Fat 25g, Carb. 24.7g, Protein 45.5g)

FRIED SALMON WITH ROMAINE LETTUCE

- *4 servings*

Ingredients

- 4 Roman Sisters
- 4 tomatoes
- 1 red onion
- 4 tablespoons white balsamic vinegar
- 6 tbsp olive oil
- Salt
- Pepper
- 400 g salmon filet (without skin)
- 1 tbsp neutral oil
- 1 bunch of chives

Preparation

Total time approx. 45min

Halve romaine lettuce in half. Quarter the tomatoes and cut into small cubes.

Dice the onion and mix together with balsamic vinegar, olive oil and diced tomatoes in a bowl. Strong with salt and pepper to taste. Mince the salmon fork-wise and fry in a pan with the oil for 90 seconds from each side. Season with salt and pepper. Tip: The salmon should still be glassy inside. Arrange lettuce hearts with the cut surface facing upwards. Distribute the salmon and drizzle everything with dressing. Cut the chives and sprinkle over the salad.

(Macros - 415kcal, protein 21g, fat 32g, carb. 8g)

SALMON WITH A MUSTARD AND LEMON NOTE

- *Servings: 2*

Ingredients

- 2 salmon fillets, approx. 200 g each
- 1/4 cup of thick cream (preferably 36%)
- 1 tablespoon Dijon mustard
- 1 tablespoon lemon juice
- 100 g cauliflower roses

Preparation

Total time approx. 30mins

Steamed the cauliflower florets and simmer in an oiled pan. Simmer for 8 minutes under low heat, covered, stirring occasionally.

In a small saucepan, fry the salmon fillets for 3 minutes on each side over low heat. Then put the salmon pan down and let it cool down.

Mix thick cream, mustard, lemon juice and add to the cooled salmon. Heat on low heat for 5 minutes.

Serve salmon prepared this way on stewed cauliflower florets

(Macros Fat 32g, Protein 36, Net carb. 1g, Calories 465)

KETO OMELETTE WITH SMOKED SALMON

- *1 serving*

Ingredients

- 30 g smoked salmon
- 1 tbsp chives fresh
- 1 teaspoon dill fresh
- 100 g eggs equal 2 pieces
- 2.5 ml of WATER
- 1/8 teaspoon salt
- 1/8 tsp pepper
- 10 g of coconut oil

Preparation

Total time approx. 15min

Wash and chop the chives and dill. The eggs with the water, salt and pepper together in a small bowl and whisk with a fork. Heat the coconut oil in a pan and add the egg mass. Reduce the temperature and let the egg slow down.

Put the smoked salmon on one half of the omelet and sprinkle the herbs over it. Fold together and serve warm.

(Macros - Calories 285, Fat 23g, Carb. 1g, Protein 20g)

SOUP RECIPES

PIZZA SOUP
- *16 serving*

Ingredients
- 300 g of passed tomatoes
- 200 g cream
- 100 g mascarpone
- 100 g red pepper
- 100 g mushrooms
- 250 g chicken cut into small pieces (mince is also possible)
- 60g salami
- 1 big onion
- 2 tbsp vegetable broth
- 250 ml of water
- 1 tbsp of olive oil available here
- Creme fraiche Cheese
- Parmesan
- Salt, pepper, oregano, black seed seeds at will

Preparation
Total time approx. 30min

Cut the onions into small cubes and fry them briefly in olive oil. Add the meat and stir fry. Season with salt and pepper. Now add the other cut vegetables (peppers, mushrooms) to the meat. Stir everything for about 5 minutes over medium heat and put everything in the vegetable broth.

The whole thing should now simmer for 10 minutes. Add the passed tomatoes, cream and mascarpone cream. Tastes of oregano, black cumin and other suitable spices. Serve the soup in a deep plate and garnish with extra creme fraiche, parmesan and fresh basil leaves.

(Macros - Calories 400, Fat 45g, Carbs 25, Proteins 7g)

MIXED VEGETABLE SOUP

- *12 servings*

Ingredients

- 500 g minced meat
- 35 g of coconut oil
- 250 g bacon (diced)
- 150 g red onion (finely diced)
- 400 g leek (cut into rings)
- 500 g broccoli (cut into small pieces)
- 500 g paprika (colorful, in stripes)
- 800 g peeled tomatoes (canned)
- 800 ml vegetable stock
- 200 g organic cream cheese double cream stage
- 300 g Kerry Gold Cheddar (finely grated)
- 35 g Dijon mustard
- 125 g gherkins (with stevia) (small cut)
- 1 tbsp erythritol
- 2 tsp locust bean gum
- Salt
- Pepper

Preparation

Total time approx. 60min

In a large pot fry the chopped onions in coconut oil. Add the minced meat and ham cubes and sauté. Season with salt and pepper, add the erythritol. Add the broth and the peeled tomatoes and simmer for 10-15 minutes.

Add leek rings, broccoli and pepper strips and simmer for another 10 minutes. Finally, stir in the cream cheese and melt the grated cheddar in the hot soup. The last whistle gets the soup with the mustard, the cucumber pieces and a last seasoning with salt and pepper. If the consistency of the soup is still too watery, mix 2 teaspoons carob seed flour with 75 ml cold water and stir into the no longer boiling soup. Bring to a boil once more - done.

(Macros - Calories 382, Carb. 8g, Protein 22g, Fat 27g)

DIETARY CAULIFLOWER SOUP WITH BACON

- *Servings: 4*

Ingredients

- large cauliflower
- 1 white onion, diced
- 1 small, chopped carrot
- 1/2 cup sour cream
- 16 slices of bacon

Preparation

Total time approx. 75mins

Divide the cauliflower into florets, put them in hot oil, add carrots and onions to them. Heat until the onion is glassy and the vegetables soft. Add 4 glasses of water and bring to a boil. Let it cook for an hour. Stir occasionally. Add cream at the end of cooking. (Harden, mixing with a little soup before pouring it into the pot.)

Fry the bacon to make it crispy. Cut into small strips and add to the soup served, sprinkling it with it so that it does not lose its crunchiness.

(Macros - Fat 19g, Protein 15g, Net carb. 5g, Calories 275)

CREAMY MUSHROOM SOUP WITH CHICKEN

- *Servings: 4*

Ingredients

- 4 cups chicken broth
- 1/2 medium onion, diced
- 350 g chopped mushrooms
- 450 g chicken thighs without skin and bones
- 3/4 cream

Preparation

Total time approx. 65mins

Cook chicken broth, onions and mushrooms on medium heat. After boiling, reduce the temperature and simmer on low heat for 30 minutes. Season with salt and pepper to taste. Fry the chicken in an oiled pan for 6 minutes on medium heat, then peel the bones and divide into shreds. Add chicken and cream to the pan, then cook for an additional 10 minutes. Finished

(Macros - Fat 23g, Protein 28g, Net carb.5g, Calories 320)

FAST KETO TOMATO SOUP
- Servings: 4

Ingredients
- 400 g Roman tomatoes
- 100 g onion, diced
- 4 tablespoons unsalted butter
- 1 cup cream
- a bunch of fresh basil

Preparation

Total time approx. 50mins

Fry the tomatoes until the crust turns red (about 5-10 minutes). During this time, occasionally rotate the pan to prevent burning. Wait for it to cool down and peel it off. In a lightly oiled pot, cook the diced onion until it becomes transparent.

Add butter, cream, 2 glasses of water and baked tomatoes, then season with salt and pepper. Cook for 20 minutes, and 5 minutes before the end add a bunch of basil. Pour into a mixer and blend until the soup is quite smooth.

(Macros - Fat 25g, Protein 2g, Net carb.5g, Calories 330)

DESSERT

SLIMMING COCKTAIL WITH COCONUT MILK AND MACADAMIA NUTS

- *Servings: 1*

Ingredients
- 2 cups unsweetened coconut milk
- 30 g macadamia nuts
- 1/4 cup unsweetened coconut flakes
- 1/2 teaspoon ground cinnamon
- 10 drops of liquid stevia

Preparation
Total time approx. 5min
Put all ingredients into the blender and mix until a creamy consistency. Sweeten with stevia to taste. If you don't like its taste, you can replace it with erythritol. Serve cold.
(Macros - Fat 38g, Protein 3g, Net carb 4g, Calories 390)

CREAMY STRAWBERRY SMOOTHIE

- *Servings: 2*

Ingredients
- Approx. 80 grams of strawberries
- 1 cup unsweetened almond or coconut milk
- 1 cup of greasy cream
- 1/2 teaspoon vanilla extract
- 10 drops of liquid stevia (optional)

Preparation
Rinse thoroughly and peel the strawberries. Pour almond or coconut milk and fatty cream into a blender. Add strawberries along with vanilla extract (and stevia if you like). Mix everything at high speed until completely combined, until a creamy consistency is obtained.
(Macros - Fat 49g, Protein 3g, Net carb 5g, Calories 430)

AVOCADO MASCARPONE SHAKE

- *1 serving*

Ingredients

- avocado
- 50 g spinach leaves
- 40 g of frozen kale
- 50 g mascarpone
- 100 g fresh organic whipped cream (at least 30% fat)
- 2 tablespoons of linseed oil
- 2 tablespoons MCT oil
- Water

Preparation

Total time approx. 15min

Slice the avocado lengthwise, remove the kernel and spoon the pulp. Put the spinach and kale together with the avocado flesh in a blender jar, add some water and mix everything. Add all other ingredients, refill with a little water and mix everything at the highest level. Finally add so much cream or water until it becomes a drinkable liquid. Alternatively, this also results in a delicious cream that can be spooned with some linseed or chia seeds.

(Macros - Calories 1292, Carb.6g, Protein 11g, Fat 134g)

LOW CARB KETO CHOCOLATE NUT CAKE

- *15 portions*

Ingredients

- 150 g Butter
- 5 Eggs
- 150 g ground almonds
- 150 g ground hazelnuts
- 2 tbsp KetoMeals LowerCarb Keto Shake Chocolate 1 tbsp approx. 10 g
- 1 packet baking powder
- 45 ml saccharin, liquid
- 1/2 bottle bitter almond aroma
- 10 g baking cocoa

Preparation

Total time approx. 55mins

Preheat oven (180° C, circulating air), line a box mold with aluminum foil. Separate the eggs and beat the egg white with 5 ml saccharin until stiff. In another bowl beat the soft butter with egg yolk, aroma and the remaining 40 ml saccharin until foamy. Add almonds, hazelnuts, Shake Chocolate, baking cocoa and baking powder and mix together.

Carefully fold in the beaten egg white and fill everything into the box form. Finish baking in the oven (50 to 60 minutes).

(Macros - Calories 265, Carb.2g, Protein 8g, Fat 23g)

A PROTEIN SHAKE WITH PEANUT BUTTER

- *Servings: 2*

Ingredients

- 2 cups unsweetened almond or coconut milk
- 62 g low-carbohydrate chocolate protein powder
- 1/4 cup peanut butter
- 2 tablespoons of coconut oil
- 10 ice cubes

Preparation

Total time approx. 5mins

Put all ingredients in the blender. Mix everything at high speed until smooth.

Tip: If you don't have chocolate flavored protein powder, you can use vanilla or unsavory protein powder instead. You also need to add 1-2 tablespoons of unsweetened cocoa powder.

(Macros - Fat 33g, Protein 33g, Net carb. 4.5g, Calories 450)

COCONUT MUFFINS WITH BLUEBERRIES

- *Servings: 1*

Ingredients

- 2 tablespoons of coconut flour
- 1/2 teaspoon baking powder
- 2 tbsp coconut oil
- 1 large egg
- 15 g fresh or frozen berries

Preparation

Total time approx. 30mins

Mix the flour and baking powder in a bowl so that there are no lumps. Add coconut oil and egg and mix thoroughly. Add berries and a pinch of salt. Transfer the dough to lightly greased muffin molds, put in the oven preheated to 180 ° C for about 18 minutes. Serve thoroughly cooled.

(Macros - Fat 33g, Protein 7g, Net carb. 5g, Calories 375)

3 WEEKS KETO MEAL PLAN

WEEK 1

DAY 1

BREAKFAST
LOW CARB SANDWICH BREAD
- *3 serving*

Ingredients
For the dough:
- 150 g almond paste (white)
- 6 organic eggs
- 50 g of coconut oil
- 30 g of xylitol (or less)
- 30 g of flax seed (crushed)
- 50 g coconut flour
- 1 teaspoon tartar baking powder (gluten-free)
- 1/2 teaspoon salt

To sprinkle:
- 10 g of flax seed (crushed)

Preparation
Total time approx. 50
Preheat the oven to 175 ° C. Melt the coconut oil and allow to cool until it is only lukewarm. Put the eggs, almond paste and coconut oil together in a blender and mix to a uniform mass.
Mix xylitol, flax seed, coconut flour, baking powder and salt in a bowl. Turn on the blender and let the dry ingredients slowly trickle to the wet mass. Continue mixing until everything is well crushed. Lay out a box tin with parchment paper, spread the dough and smooth it out. Bake 35-40 minutes.
(Macros – Calorie 359, carb 7.5g (Net carb 2.5g), protein 15g, fat 28.3g)

LUNCH
BEETROOT SKEWERS WITH GORGONZOLA AND WALNUTS

- *serving*

Ingredients

- 185 g of Gorgonzola
- 135 g beetroot pre-cooked
- 15 g of walnuts

Preparation

Total time approx. 15min

If you use raw beetroot, you have to cook and peel it first. It is recommended that you pre-cooked beetroot. Roll the gorgonzola and beetroot. Arrange both alternately on toothpicks. Serve the skewers with the walnuts. So easy and fast you are done.
(Macros – Calories 788, 64.1 g fat, 12.0g net carb.), 42.0g protein)

DINNER
LOW CARB RISOTTO WITH GOAT CREAM CHEESE (DINNER)

- *3 serving*

Ingredients

- 200 g of cauliflower
- 100 g mushrooms
- 65 g cocktail tomatoes
- 1 small shallot
- 35 g of pasture butter
- 100 ml vegetable stock
- 55 g of Parmesan
- 1 pinch of freshly ground pepper
- 65 g goat cream cheese
- Arugula leaves
- Chives

Preparation

Total time approx. 30

Wash the vegetables. Divide the cauliflower into florets. Gradually process the florets in the blender into rice-grain-sized pieces. To do this, always put just a handful of cauliflower in the blender at once. Slice the mushrooms, quarter the tomatoes. Peel the shallot and finely chop it.

Omit half of the butter in a pan, lightly brown the shallot in it and add the cauliflower rice. Braise for 2 minutes.

Pour the vegetable stock and cook the cauliflower in it for about 5-8 minutes until the water is completely evaporated. Rub the parmesan and stir in the risotto. Season well with salt and pepper. Fry the mushrooms in the remaining butter. Arrange the risotto with fried mushrooms and tomatoes and refine with the goat's cheese. Wash the chives and rucola leaves, shake dry, cut the chives into small rolls. Then decorate the risotto with it.

(Macros – Calories 640, carb.12g, protein 32g, fat 52g)

DAY 2

BREAKFAST
BREAKFAST-LIZZA: LOW CARB PIZZA WITH BACON AND FRIED EGG

- *2 serving*

Ingredients

- fresh pizza dough
- 50 g Brie
- 2 tablespoons green pesto
- 2 tablespoons bacon cubes
- 2 eggs
- Salt
- Pepper
- 2 stalks of fresh basil

Preparation

Total time approx. 45min

Preheat the oven to 200 degrees. Place the dough on a baking sheet covered with baking paper and prick several times with a fork. Bake in the hot oven for 5 minutes, then remove from the oven.

Roll the brie. Spread the pesto on top of the pizza dough and spread the pieces of pancake and bacon. Put in the oven again for 2-3 minutes, so that the cheese runs smoothly.

Beat the eggs and let them slide gently on the pizza. Bake in the oven for about 7 more minutes until the eggs have the desired degree of cooking.

Remove from the oven, season with salt and pepper and garnish with the fresh basil leaves.
(Macros - 373kcal, protein 26g, fat 25g, carb. 4g)

LUNCH
CESAR SALAD WITH LOW CARB CROUTONS
- *1 serving*

Ingredients
- slice Bread Fit baking
- 15 g of butter from pasture milk
- 2 slices of bacon
- 10 g ghee made from willow butter
- 125 g chicken breast fillets
- 30 g of Parmesan
- 75 g of Romana salad
- 125 g cucumber
- 35 g of celery
- 1 tsp mustard
- 1 tbsp olive oil
- 1 tablespoon of apple cider vinegar
- Salt and pepper

Preparation
Total time approx. 40min

The Bread Fit can be prepared according to the instructions on the tin. You only need one slice of it this time - but you can also freeze the low carb bread very well. If you then toast it fresh, you always have delicious, fresh bread.

Cut the slice Bread Fit into even, small cubes. Drain the butter in a pan and fry the bread cubes into crispy croutons. Then take the croutons out of the pan and put them aside for a moment.

Now put the bacon slices in the pan and fry them slowly until crisp. Take it from the pan and put it aside. Put the ghee in the pan and heat it. In it, the chicken breast is seared from both sides. Then you let it fry in the hot pan until it is cooked. In the meantime, you can wash the salad and pluck it into bite-sized pieces. Put the salad in a salad bowl.

Brush the cucumber and celery. The cucumber can be cut in half lengthwise and cut into slices, the celery as well. Give the vegetables to the salad. From mustard, apple cider vinegar, olive oil, salt and pepper you stir a dressing together. Mix this dressing under the salad in the bowl.

Now you can cut the finished chicken breast into slices and drape on the salad. You can also cut the bacon a bit and put it on the salad. Finally, top the salad with Parmesan shavings and the low carb croutons.

(Macros – Calories 691, 49.4g fat, 7.4g net carb, 51.4g protein)

<u>DINNER</u>
CAMEMBERT IN BACON COAT

- *2 serving*

Ingredients

- 2 rolls of goat camembert (100g)
- 100 g bacon (nitrate-free)
- 100 g of pickle salad
- 2 tbsp balsamic vinegar
- 2 tablespoons MCT oil
- Himalayan salt

Preparation

Total time approx. 30min

Wrap each camembert well with 50 g bacon. Heat a pan on a mild heat. Put the wrapped camembert into it and slowly let the fat melt out of the bacon. Once there is enough fat in the pan, raise the temperature slightly and brown the bacon nicely in your own fat. Serve together with fresh salad. Drizzle with balsamic and MCT oil and season with a little Himalaya salt.

(Macros – Calories 690, 4g carb. 31g protein, 60g fat)

DAY 3

BREAKFAST
THAI BREAKFAST OMELETTE

- *4 serving*

Ingredients

- 8 eggs
- 4 tablespoons fish sauce
- 0.5 bunch cilantro
- 4 spring onions
- 1 red pepper
- 4 tbsp oil

Preparation

Total time approx. 15min

Whisk eggs in a bowl. Stir in the fish sauce.
Wash cilantro, shake dry and chop. Wash the spring onions and cut into fine rings. Wash the peppers and cut into very fine strips. Put everything under the egg mass.
Heat 1 tbsp of oil in the pan. Pour one-fourth of the egg mixture into the pan, let it stand, turn it over and fry it from the other side. Bake 3 more omelets in this way.
(Macros - 302kcal, protein 16g, fat 23g, carb. 7g)

LUNCH
LUNCH CHICKEN SAUSAGES

- *1 serving*

Ingredients

- 3 large eggs
- 1 chicken sausage, cut into bite-size
- 1/3 cup broccoli, chopped
- 1 cup chopped spinach
- 1 tablespoon herb-fed butter
- 1-ounce goat cheese, crumbled
- ½ medium avocado, sliced

Preparation
Total time approx. 15mins
In a small bowl, beat the eggs. In a large saucepan over medium heat, melt the butter. Sauté the broccoli until tender, about 5 minutes. Add eggs, sausages and spinach. Stir the eggs until well cooked, about 5 minutes.
Place on a plate, garnish with goat cheese, avocado and let cool a few minutes, enjoy.
(Macros - Calories 690, fat 55g, 13g of carb. (6g of net carb.), protein 39g)

DINNER
SHRIMP ALFREDO
- *4 Servings*

Ingredients
- lb. shrimp, cleaned and peeled
- 120g cream cheese, cubed
- ½ cup parmesan, grated
- ½ cup whole milk
- ¼ cup kale
- 1 tablespoon butter, salted
- 1 tablespoon garlic powder
- 1 teaspoon basil
- 1 teaspoon salt
- 5 whole sun-dried tomatoes, sliced
- 1 pack zucchini noodles for serving

Preparation
Total time approx. 30mins
Melt the butter in a pan and add the shrimp. Cook the shrimp until they are pink. Add cream cheese and milk. Stir until melted and creamy. Add the garlic powder, basil, salt and Parmesan cheese. Stir until they are melted. Stir in tomatoes and kale
Serve on zucchini noodles
(Macros - Calories 297, Fat 17g, Carb.6g, Protein 22g)

DAY 4

BREAKFAST
BREAKFAST LASAGNA

- *12 servings*

Ingredients

- 900 g of eggs
- 40 g of butter
- 400 g sausage coarse
- 400 g cream cheese
- 350 ml beef broth
- 100 g cooked ham
- 100 g bacon
- 125 g of grated Parmesan
- 125 g Mozzarella
- 1 tsp salt
- 1/2 tsp pepper

Preparation

Total time approx. 1hr 15min

Preheat the oven to 160 °. Grease a large pan well and let it get hot on the stove. Whisk all eggs in a large bowl and pour half into the pan. Now let it falter like an omelet. After about 4 minutes, reduce the heat. Season with salt and pepper. A turn is not necessary. Do the same with the rest of the egg mass. First set aside. Press the sausage meat out of the peel and place in a pan. Approximately roast crumbly for 5-6 min. Then stir in the cream cheese and add the broth. Simmer the sauce with constant stirring for 2 minutes until it thickens. Season with salt and pepper. Now grease a square, high casserole dish and add the first layer of the canned egg mass. Spread the bratwurst sauce on top and top with the cooked ham. Fill in the second layer of egg and again spread a portion of the sauce on it. Cover with the ham and the sliced mozzarella. Add the remaining sauce and sprinkle with Parmesan cheese. Bake in the oven for 30 min at 160 ° C.

(Macros - Calories 393, Fat 31g, Carb. 2g, Protein 26g)

LUNCH
THIN-SKINNED WILLOW OX WITH STRAWBERRY AND HUGO SALAD

- *2 servings*

Ingredients

- 4 thin ox shreds
- 60 g of cut salad
- 2 stalks of apple mint
- 1/2 turnip
- 200 g strawberries
- 2 tablespoons of elderflower vinegar
- 4 tablespoons of olive oil or MCT oil
- 1 tablespoon of ghee for frying

For marinating:

- Apple mint
- 2 tablespoons of olive oil or MCT oil
- Salt
- Pepper
- Paprika powder, sweet

Preparation

Total time approx. 2h

Mix oil, mint and spices, rub the meat with it and let it rest for a few hours. Wash the lettuce and the mint and spin dry. Wash, clean and slice the strawberries. Peel the whitefish and finely dice it. Chop the mint. Mix the salad with the mint and arrange on a plate or in a decorative salad bowl. Sprinkle strawberries and turnips over it. For the dressing, mix the elderflower vinegar with salt and pepper and stir in the olive oil. Just before serving, pour over the salad. Now throw the pieces of ox on the grill for a short time or fry them briefly from both sides in a pan in ghee.

(Macros – Calorie 598, 24.3g protein, 9.7g carb, 46.9g fat)

DINNER
CAULIFLOWER PUREE WITH TURKEY BREAST FILLET AND LAMB'S LETTUCE

- *2 serving*

Ingredients

- 500 g of cauliflower
- 50 ml of cream
- 1 tbsp butter
- Pinch (s) of nutmeg
- 0.5 tsp salt
- 2 Turkey fillets
- 0.5 tsp paprika sweet
- 0.5 teaspoon paprika rosenscharf
- 2 tablespoons rapeseed oil
- 100 g corn salad
- 1 shallot
- 2 tablespoons apple cider vinegar
- 3 tbsp olive oil
- Pepper (fresh)

Preparation

Total time approx. 45min

Wash cauliflower and cut into small pieces. Then cook in salted water for 20 minutes. Meanwhile wash and pluck salad. Peel the shallot and cut into fine cubes. Put both in a salad bowl. Season the turkey breasts with paprika, pepper and salt. Heat the rapeseed oil in a pan, sauté the turkey breasts and fry for 5-6 minutes on each side over medium heat. Drain cauliflower and finely stomp with a potato masher. Possibly. purée a little more finely with a blender. Add the butter, cream and nutmeg and whisk the mixture creamy with a whisk. Salad with apple cider vinegar, olive oil, pepper and salt. Serve with turkey breast and cauliflower puree.

(Macros - 683kcal, protein 38g, fat 54g, carb. 8g)

DAY 5

BREAKFAST
SANDWICH FOR BREAKFAST
- *2 serving*

Ingredients
- 5 pcs. Egg
- 120 g Cream cheese
- 1 tbsp. a spoon Erythritol
- 70 g Almond flour
- ½ teaspoon Baking powder
- Salt
- 3 tbsp. spoons Butter
- 2 pcs Cutlets
- 4 pc Bacon slice
- 2 pcs Cheddar Cheese Slice

Preparation
Total time approx. 25min
In a large bowl, beat with a mixer 2 eggs and cream cheese until lush. Add almond flour, baking powder and salt, mix until smooth. Put a tablespoon of oil in a pan and put on medium heat. After it melts, fry four pancakes. Cook for 1-2 minutes on each side until the edges rise and it will be easy to turn them over. Fry for another 2-3 minutes until tender. Leave them warm while you cook the patties, bacon and eggs. Beat three eggs lightly, pour half into a preheated pan, and fry. Fry meatballs and bacon. Collect the sandwich: put the finished cutlet on the pancake, on top of the egg, bacon, cheese and pancake again.
(Macros - Calories 525, Fat 46g, Carb. 6g, Protein 25g)

LUNCH
GAUCHO KETO BURGER
- *4 servings*

Ingredients
Patty's
- 450 g ground beef
- 250 g sausage meat (the inside of a sausage)

- Chopped 30 g of shallots
- 5 g garlic clove

- 1/4 tsp pepper black
- 1 tsp salt

Egg Salad
- 200 g fried egg 1 fried egg
- 100 g lettuce 1 large lettuce

Sauce:
- 100 ml burger pesto

Preparation

Total time approx. 30min

Mix all Pattie ingredients and shape into patties with a hamburger press

The patties on a grill min. Fry for 15 minutes Heat a greased frying pan on the grill, place the egg shaper in the pan, add an egg and finish cooking.

Put patties on lettuce leaves, put the egg on top and add the burger pesto. Finished is the Gaucho Keto Burger.

(Macros - Calories 618, Fat 50g, Carb. 7g, Protein 42g)

DINNER
COD WITH MACADAMIA CRUST

- *2 servings*

Ingredients

- 2 cod fillets (125g)
- 50 g of macadamia
- 1egg
- 2 zucchini (200g, green or yellow)
- 38 g coconut oil (2 tbsp + 1 heaped tsp)

Preparation

Total time approx. 40min

Finely chop the macadamia with a large knife and place in a deep plate. Whisk the egg in a deep plate. Dab the cod fillets and turn in the egg. Then turn into the chopped macadamia until the fillets are well covered. Slightly press the breading gently. Heat half of the coconut oil in a pan. Whether it's hot enough, you can easily test: You push the top of a wooden cooking spoon into it. If it

begins to sizzle at this point, the oil is hot enough. Add the breaded fish fillets and sauté on both sides until golden brown. Be careful when turning so that the crust does not break. Cut the zucchini diagonally into thin slices. Heat the remaining coconut oil and brown the zucchini. Sprinkle with coarse sea salt.
(Macros – Calories 531, 6.5g carb., 28.5g protein. 42g fat)

DAY 6

BREAKFAST
STUFFED AVOCADO WITH EGG
- *2 servings*

Ingredients
- 1 avocado
- 2 eggs
- Salt
- Pepper

Preparation
Total time approx. 25min
Preheat the oven to 180°C (circulating air). Halve and core avocado.
Put avocado halves in a casserole dish. Pour 1 egg into each half and fill in the core of the avocado and season with pepper and salt. Bake for 20 minutes, decorate and serve.
(Macros - Calories 204, Fat 20g, Carb. 4g, Protein 7g)

LUNCH
SZEGED GOULASH
- *2 servings*

Ingredients
- 250 g pork shoulder
- 300 g sauerkraut
- 1 small onion (finely chopped)
- 20 g of ghee (or coconut oil)
- 1 tablespoon tomato paste
- 1 TL paprika
- Soup (or water)
- Salt
- 1 tbsp marjoram

- 1 toe garlic (finely chopped)
- Caraway (whole)
- Bay leaf
- 3-4 tablespoons sour cream

Preparation

Total time approx. 50min

Roast the onions in golden ghee until golden. Stir in pork shoulder, reduce heat and add paprika powder. Add warm soup or water. Heat again, season with salt, pepper, caraway, bay leaf and garlic and cook well covered.

Reduce heat and add the diced raw meat and sauerkraut. Slowly simmer for about 45 minutes on a low heat until the sauerkraut and meat are tender.

Finally, refine with sour cream.

(Macros - Calories 398, Carb. 5g, Protein 24g, Fat 25g)

DINNER
RADISH NOODLES WITH ROCKET PESTO

- *1 serving*

Ingredients

- 1 radish (white)
- 150 g of rocket
- 25 g sunflower seeds
- 5 tbsp olive oil
- 2 tablespoons of ghee
- Salt

Preparation

Total time approx. 20min

Pesto: Wash the rocket and pat dry. Roast the sunflower seeds in a larger pan (without fat!). We need the big pan again. Chop the kernels in a blender, add rocket and olive oil and chop everything until a fine, creamy pesto mass is produced. Season with salt.

Radish noodles: Process the radish into noodles with a spiral cutter or a peeler. Fry the radish noodles in the pan with the ghee for a short time. Stir in the pesto and spread well, heat briefly and then serve.

(Macros - Calories 468, Carb. 6g, Protein 6g, Fat 44g)

DAY 7

BREAKFAST
CRACKER IN BACON DRESSING GOWN

- *1 serving*

Ingredients
- 1 cracker
- 1 slice of Gouda
- 100 g bacon (in strips)

Preparation
Total time approx. 15min

Cut the cracker lengthwise in the middle. Slice the cheese into long strips and cover one half with it. As thick as you want it to be.

Then you put the second half of the hamburger on the cheese and wrap the whole thing with the bacon. So, everything stays stable and does not slip. Then the wrapped Knacker comes for 15 minutes at about 160 ° C in the oven. For urgent: for 2-3 minutes in the microwave grill.

(Macros - Calories 716, Carb.2g, Protein 42g, Fat 59g)

LUNCH
SALAD WRAPS

- *4 Servings*

Ingredients

SALAD
- 300 g of salad
- 150 g of cucumber

DRESSING
- 110 g breakfast bacon
- 200 g mushrooms
- 60 ml of chicken broth
- 10 ml coconut vinegar
- 10 ml of oil
- 2 tablespoons of parsley
- 1/2 tsp Stevia liquid
- 1/2 teaspoon salt
- 1/4 tsp pepper

FILLING

- 500 g minced meat
- 80 g onion
- 7 g garlic
- 4 ml of Coconut Amino
- 1/4 tsp fish sauce
- 10 g ginger fresh
- 10 g spring onion
- 5 ml coconut vinegar

Preparation

Total time approx. 40min

Dressing

Cut the bacon into 1cm pieces and fry in a pan until crispy in the oil. Cut the mushrooms into small pieces and add to the bacon. Roast 5 minutes together.

Add vinegar and broth and simmer for another 5 min. Stir in salt, pepper and stevia. Sprinkle with parsley and set aside.

Filling:

Fry the minced meat in a pan and then remove with a ladle. The liquid should remain in the pan. Chop the onion and garlic, grate the ginger and fry everything in the pan.

Add vinegar, coconut amino and the fish sauce. Add the minced meat and spring onion.

Salad:

Wash the lettuce and pick the leaves from the stalk. Serve on a plate. Distribute the minced meat mixture evenly on the lettuce leaves and add the dressing. Add the cucumber to taste.

(Macros - Calories 434, Fat 31g, Carbohydrates 6g, Protein 33g)

DINNER

TURKEY SALTIMBOCCA WITH BROCCOLI

- *4 serving*

Ingredients

- 8 leaves of sage
- 4 narrow flat turkey schnitzel
- 8 slice (s) of Black Forest ham
- 2 tbsp sunflower oil
- 1 clove of garlic
- 1 teaspoon flour
- Salt
- Pepper
- 350 ml whole milk
- Grated 100 g Emmental
- Grated nutmeg

- 1 teaspoon lemon juice
- 600 g of broccoli

Preparation

Total time approx. 25min

Wash sage and pat dry. Wash schnitzel, pat dry and cut in half. Tap very thinly between the layers of the freezer bag and lightly season with salt and pepper. Cover each schnitzel with 1 sage of sage and 1 slice of ham and stick with wooden skewers.

Wash broccoli, clean and divide into florets. Cook in boiling salted water for about 4 minutes, drain and keep warm. Heat 2 tablespoons of oil in a large pan and fry the meat for about 6 minutes while turning. Peel garlic and chop finely. Heat 1 teaspoon of oil in a saucepan, sauté garlic in it for a short time. Dust with flour and sauté briefly while stirring. Deglaze with milk and simmer for 2-3 minutes. Add the cheese and melt over low heat while stirring. Season the sauce with salt, nutmeg and lemon juice, froth briefly with the blender. Arrange meat, broccoli and sauce on plates, sprinkle with pepper.

(Macros - 547kcal, protein 57g, fat 30g, carb 15g)

WEEK 2
DAY 1

BREAKFAST
NUT CEREAL

- 4 servings

Ingredients

- 200 g of nuts ((which you like, e.g. hazelnuts, almonds, pecans, walnuts))
- 80 grams of grated coconut
- 2 tablespoons of flaxseed
- 50 g sunflower seeds
- 1 tsp vanilla powder
- 2 teaspoons cinnamon
- 2 tablespoons Xucker light (if really necessary)

Preparation

Total time approx. 35min

Preheat the oven to 100 ° C. Coarsely chop the nuts and mix with the grated coconut, linseeds and sunflower seeds. Spread the mixture on a baking sheet lined with baking paper and sprinkle with cinnamon and vanilla. (And the Xucker, if you really need it). Push the baking tray into the oven for about 30 minutes.

Every 10 minutes you should stir the mixture roughly, so that the cereal is nicely browned from all sides. Let the cereal then cool before you eat it. Filled everything in a jar and tightly closed, so it lasts a long time.

(Macros - Calories 545, Carb. 8g, Protein 14g, Fat 49g)

LUNCH
CHEESE & MINCE AND LEEK PAN

- 4 servings

Ingredients

- tbsp coconut oil
- 500 g minced meat
- 2 rods leek
- 1 onion (red)
- 1 toe garlic
- 600 ml broth

- 200 g processed cheese
- Pepper
- Salt
- Caraway seed
- Nutmeg

Preparation

Total time approx. 15mins

Fry the minced meat in a large and high pan with the onions and garlic. Cut the leek into rolls and fry these with the hack. Erase everything with the broth. Add the melted cheese and let it simmer briefly. Spice everything well and serve.

(Macros - Calories 526, Carb. 4g, Protein 35g, Fat 41g)

DINNER
CAULIFLOWER PAN

- *2 servings*

Ingredients

- Cauliflower
- 1 medium red onion
- 1 pepper (orange)
- 5 tablespoons of coconut oil
- 3 tablespoons parsley (minced)
- 5 tbsp Parmesan (finely grated)
- 50 g (willow) butter
- Salt
- Pepper
- Chili (if you like it hot)

Preparation

Total time approx. 30mins

Cut the onions into thin slices. Wash the peppers and cut into cubes. Divide the cauliflower into florets, wash well and drain. Cut 5mm thick slices. In a wok or a large pan, heat the coconut oil, add the cauliflower and fry well with constant stirring. (About 7-8 minutes). Then add the onions and fry for another 2-3 minutes until the onions soften slightly. Add the paprika cubes and fry for another 2-3 minutes, stirring constantly, turning the whole mixture. Add the butter, melt and season with salt, pepper and if you like chili to taste. Fry for another 2-3 minutes until the cauliflower is well and still bite-resistant, then you can take the pan off the stove. Add the finely chopped parsley and grated Parmesan cheese, stir well and melt the cheese.

Serve warm, garnish with parsley and parmesan.
(Macros - Calories 638, Carb.11g, Protein 9g, Fat 57g)

DAY 2

BREAKFAST
EGGS HACK PAN

- *1 serving*

Ingredients

- 2 eggs
- 1 tomato (about 50g)
- 50 g of paprika (about half a yellow pepper)
- 30 g pine nuts
- 30 g minced meat
- 30 g of coconut oil

Preparation

Total time approx. 15min

Brown the pine nuts in a pan with a little coconut oil. Dice the tomatoes and add them to the pan with the minced meat. If the minced meat is well-fried, add the 2 eggs and fry until finished. Season as needed with salt, pepper and other spices.
(Macros - Calories 758, Carb. 10g, Protein 26g, Fat 65g)

LUNCH
BACON BURGER ROLL

- *1 serving*

Ingredients

- 900 g minced meat
- 2 eggs
- 2 teaspoons salt
- 1 tsp pepper
- Granulated 2 teaspoons of garlic
- 6 slices of ham
- 8-10 slices of Kerry Gold Cheddar
- 2 packs. Bacon
- 1 pepper
- 5 small tomatoes

Preparation

Total time approx. 60min

Preheat the oven to 180 ° C. Mix the minced meat, eggs and spices well, spread on a tin foil lined with olive oil like a pizza dough. Place the ham and cheese slices on top and then evenly on top. Wash the peppers and tomatoes, dice and spread on the cheese, now carefully roll in the mincemeat while not rolling up the aluminum foil. On a second aluminum foil, place the bacon strips close together. Place the chopping roll on it and roll it up so that the bacon strips completely surround the chopping roll. Wrap everything together with aluminum foil and close it so that nothing can run out. Bake in the oven for 25 minutes. After these 25 minutes, remove the aluminum foil, set the oven to 260 ° C and bake for another 20 minutes. Let cool for 5 minutes and serve with a little salad or other side dish.
(Macros - Calories 941, Carb. 3g, Protein 76g, Fat 67g)

DINNER
MUSHROOMS WITH BOLOGNESE AND FETA
- *1 serving*

Ingredients
Bolognese
- 20 g olive oil (or coconut oil)
- 1 shallot
- 60 g of beef
- 150 g of tomato
- 15 g of tomato paste
- Salt
- Pepper
- Paprika
- Chili
- Italian herbs
- 2 tsp Sambal Oelek

Filled mushrooms
- 50 g feta cheese 45% fat
- 200 g Portobello mushrooms
- 25 g goat cream cheese

Preparation
Total time approx. 45min
Bolognese:
Heat the olive oil in a saucepan, dice the shallot into small pieces and fry in a glass. Add the minced meat and sauté. Cut the fresh tomatoes into small cubes, add to the saucepan and cook

everything at low speed. Season with Italian herbs, salt, pepper, paprika and / or chili and Sambal Oelek. Add the tomato puree and season to taste. Simmer until the sauce is relatively sticky and the liquid has evaporated.

Filled mushrooms:

Dice feta cheese. Unscrew the Portobello mushroom stalk and cut into small cubes. Use a spoon to scrape out the mushrooms to make a nice hollow and to have enough stuffing. The scratched, the stems and the feta under the Bolognese lift. Split the Bolognese on all mushrooms and fill the mushrooms with it. Rub the goat's cheese and spread over it. Bake circulating air at approx. 180 ° C for approx. 30 minutes in the middle of the oven. The mushrooms are ready when they are shriveled.

(Macros - Calories 573, Carb. 5g, Protein 27g, Fat 40g)

DAY 3

BREAKFAST
KETO CRISPBREAD

- *20 servings*

Ingredients

- 50 g sunflower seeds
- 50 g pumpkin seeds
- 30 g of flaxseed
- 50 g of sesame seeds
- 2 tablespoons psyllium husk
- 200 ml of water
- 1/2 teaspoon salt

Preparation

Total time approx. 1hr 15min

Preheat the oven to 150 ° C convection. Put the ingredients in a bowl, mix well and let the dough rest for about 15 minutes in a smooth, smooth mass. If the mixture is too firm, add some more water. Lay out a baking tray with baking paper or a baking mat and spread the mixture as thin as possible on the plate. Please make sure that there are no holes and the dough is not too thick. Put the baking tray in the oven for about 60 minutes and bake the crispbread so that it is lightly browned and crispy. Let the baking

sheet cool down before you break off the crispbread and break it into pieces.
In an airtight container you can keep the crispbread very well for a while, they will stay crispy.
(Macros - Calories 51, Carb. 1g, Protein 2g, Fat 4g)

LUNCH
SUSHI
- *1 Serving*

Ingredients
- 150 g of cauliflower
- Sesame oil
- 3 g apple cider vinegar
- 15 g cream cheese
- Salt
- Nori
- Cucumber (small stripes)
- Carrots (small stripes)
- Avocado (hate) (small stripes)
- Organic smoked salmon

Preparation
Total time approx. 20mins
Finely chop the cauliflower and fry in a frying pan with sesame oil for about 5-10 minutes, so that it still has some bite. Let cool down. Mix cider vinegar with cream cheese and a little salt and then mix with the cauliflower rice. Spread the cauliflower mixture thinly on a Noori leaf, leaving 2 cm above the top. Cover with a slice of cucumber, carrot, avocado and fresh raw salmon, roll in tightly and cut into 1cm thick rolls.
(Macros - Calories 503, Carb. 6g, Protein 10g, Fat 46g)

DINNER
ROAST TURKEY ROLL
- *8 servings*

Ingredients
- kg turkey breast
- 4 peppers (2 each red and yellow)
- 2 tbsp olive oil
- 100 g bacon (or bacon)
- 125 ml broth
- 70 g Gouda (ideally aged for 12 months)
- 4 tablespoons of basil (fresh)
- 100 g (willow) butter
- 50 g of coconut oil
- Salt
- Pepper
- 1 pound of bacon (about 8 slices)

Preparation

Total time approx. 2hrs 10min

Prepare meat: Either you already buy a ready-sliced turkey breast or cut it yourself to a large plate. Put some cling film on the meat and gently beat the meat with a meat tenderizer. Remove the foil and season both sides vigorously with salt and pepper.

Prepare filling: Wash the peppers, core them and cut them into small cubes. Really not too big, otherwise it will not roll later. Steam the chili cubes in hot oil (ghee or coconut oil) for about 5 minutes. Cut the bacon / bacon into small cubes and place in a large bowl. Grate the well matured cheese, preferably coarse, not too fine. Add the cheese to the bacon cubes in the bowl. Cut up so much fresh basil into small strips until you have about 4 tablespoons and add the herbs along with about half of the steamed paprika cubes to the large bowl of the other ingredients. Salt and pepper the whole mixture, add the olive oil and stir well.

Fill and fry: Preheat the oven to about 180 ° C top / bottom heat. Spread the bacon-cheese-basil-pepper-mixture evenly on the meat-plate, smooth everything and roll the meat carefully. Make sure you do not tear the meat.

Then wrap kitchen string around the roll (see instructions below). In a roasting pan, heat the coconut oil and about 50g of butter, and fry the turkey roll in it from all sides over medium heat for about 5 minutes. Now distribute the remaining pepper cubes around the roast and cover it with the remaining butter. Lay the bacon slices on top to prevent the roast from burning and becoming juicy. Now put the prepared roast turkey on the middle rail in the preheated oven. Approximately Fry open for 30 minutes. Then add the broth to the gravy, fry the meat open again for 30 minutes, more often (so every 5-10 minutes) with gravy over. Cover the roast (with aluminum foil or the lid of the roasting pan, for example) and fry for another 30 minutes. Take the roast out of the oven after these 90 minutes, remove the cooking thread and let the roast rest for 5-10 minutes.

You can now puree the gravy, including the pepper cubes, etc., which results in a tasty gravy. If necessary, add a little more basil and season to taste. Slice the turkey roast about 3cm wide and serve with the sauce.

(Macros - Calories 409, Carb. 5g, Protein 35g, Fat 26g)

DAY 4

BREAKFAST
MASCARPONE PANCAKES
- 4 Servings

Ingredients
- 100 g mascarpone
- 50 g almonds (ground)
- 3 egg
- Vanilla Xucker
- 1/2 teaspoon baking powder

Preparation

Total time approx. 10min

The preparation is also very simple. Mix all ingredients well and fry in coconut oil in a small pan. Then just whip cream until stiff and spread on a pancake. Either curl up or plaster the same way.

(Macros - Calories 250, Carb. 2g, Protein 10g, Fat 21g)

LUNCH
SPICY MINCE CASSEROLE WITH CAULIFLOWER
- *6 serving*

Ingredients
- celery (about 700g)
- 200 g parsley (fresh)
- 200 g of mint (fresh, or 1 heaped tablespoon of dried mint)
- 500 g lamb meat (also with bone)
- 1 onion (big)
- 1 tsp turmeric
- 1/2 tsp saffron (ground)
- 2 tablespoons of lemon juice
- 75 g (willow) butter
- 60 g of ghee (or more)

Preparation
Total time approx. 2 hours 20 minutes

If you use fresh herbs: Wash the fresh herbs, free them from the stems and chop the leaves small. Put some ghee in a pan and fry the fresh herbs for about 20 minutes, stirring constantly. They must not turn black. Put the herbs aside. If you use dried herbs, skip this step.

Cut the onions into small cubes and add to the herbs. Fry in medium heat in a large pan, pot or wok in a little ghee until golden brown. Spread turmeric over the onions and turn everything around. Cut the meat into pieces about 2x2cm in size. Put the meat in the pan and fry for about 8-10 minutes. The meat should then be lightly browned all around. So that the sauce gets an additional flavor, you can still add the bones of the meat, if you have any. Add saffron over the meat and season well with pepper. Clean celery and cut into pieces about 2cm long. Now add the fried (or dried) herbs and celery to the meat and stir well. Pour about half a liter of water, stir well, and let it simmer for about 1.5 hours on a low heat (lid on top). After the meat has cooked for about an hour, salt everything and stir in the lemon juice and butter. If the water in the pot / in the wok becomes too small, add a little cold water. However, it should evaporate as little water as possible. Serve everything with cauliflower rice.

(Macros - Calories 431, Carb.10g, Protein 30g, Fat 28g)

DINNER
BROCCOLI CHEDDAR SOUP

- *4 servings*

Ingredients

- 30 g (willow) butter
- 30 g red onion (chopped)
- 1 garlic (toe, grated)
- 700 ml chicken broth
- 1 broccoli (about 500g)
- 1 tbsp. Parmesan
- 100 g organic whipped cream at least 30% fat
- 120 g Kerrygold Cheddar (grated)
- 1/2 tsp. Xanthan gum
- 2 slices of bacon (optional)
- Salt
- Pepper

Preparation

Total time approx. 30min

Chop the onions and rub or squeeze the garlic clove. Add the onion and garlic and butter to a large pot and sauté over medium heat. Cut broccoli into small florets and add to the pot with the chicken broth. Simmer over medium heat until broccoli is tender. Season the soup with salt, pepper and other spices to taste. Add the cream, parmesan and cheddar, stir well until everything has melted. To bind the soup, add some xanthan gum and stir well again to avoid lumps. If desired, serve the soup with chopped bacon - but you can also omit it.

(Macros - Calories 303, Carb. 4g, Protein 13g, Fat 24g)

DAY 5

BREAKFAST
OOPSIE SANDWICH ROLLS

- *4 pieces*

Ingredients

- 4 eggs
- 150 g organic cream cheese double cream stage
- 1 pinch of salt

Preparation

Total time approx. 30min

Preheat the oven to 150 ° C (top and bottom heat). Beat up the eggs and separate. Beat the egg whites stiff - the stiffer the better. Pay attention to a fat-free bowl, etc., otherwise it will not work. Possibly. Also helps a small pinch of salt, so that the protein is stiff. Mix in another bowl of egg yolk and cream cheese to a smooth mass. The egg whites are now carefully lifted in the yolk and cream cheese mixture. Add a pinch of salt and spread the dough with a spoon evenly on the baking sheet lined with baking paper. Four servings for larger oopsies, six servings for smaller oopsies. The oopsies are now baked at 150 ° C for about 25 minutes. After baking, the oopsies can still be sprinkled with sesame or other spices. Allow it to cool well before eating.

(Macros - Calories 197, Carb. 1g, Protein 10g, Fat 16g)

LUNCH
KETOGENIC PIZZA

- *8 pieces*

Ingredients

- 45 g almond flour (partially oiled, light, finely ground)
- 20 g of egg white powder
- 15 g gold flour (finely ground)
- 10 g psyllium husk (finely ground)
- 10 g citrus fiber
- 10 g of baking powder
- 1/4 tsp salt
- 175 ml of water

- 1/4 tsp guar gum (optional)
- Bamboo fiber (to roll out)

Preparation

Total time approx. 15min

Preheat the oven to 250 ° C. Mix all ingredients (except bamboo fibers) well. Knead the dough well with damp hands and form a round flat cake. Brush the work surface with bamboo fiber and roll out the pizza dough to the desired size. If necessary, turn several times and lightly rinse several times with bamboo fiber. Place the pizza dough on the round pizza plate or on a baking tray designed several times with baking paper. Prove the pizza now according to your wishes. Ideally, all the ingredients are already prepared, the longer he stands with sauce, the stickier he gets. Brush the pizza completely with tomato paste, not too thick, otherwise the dough stays soft. Give it herbs and spices to taste, it is usually a mixture of Italian herbs. One part of the pizza is covered with salami, another part with ham. As a cheese, a mixture of Emmental, Edam and Mozzarella has proven, but there is every taste different. Place the pizza tray in the preheated oven and bake at 250 ° C for about 8-12 minutes. The duration depends on the oven and on the amount of toppings on the pizza. Bake the pizza until the rim is brown and the cheese has run dry. After baking, place the pizza on a wire rack to cool it down, making the bottom crispy again.

(Macros - Calories 55, Carb. 1g, Protein 4g, Fat 3g)

DINNER
GRATINATE AVOCADO

- *1 serving*

Ingredients

- 1 avocado (hate)
- 2 small tomatoes
- 50 g bacon
- 30 g (willow) butter
- 75 g Gouda

Preparation

Total time approx. 20min

Halve the avocado, remove the kernel, cut the pulp into small pieces. Dice the tomatoes and the bacon, put everything together with the butter in an ovenproof dish. Sprinkle the cheese over and bake everything at 180 ° C circulating air for about 15 minutes to the desired tan.
(Macros - Calories 1063, Carb. 2g, Protein 28g, Fat 102g)

DAY 6

BREAKFAST
LOOSE AND CINNAMON PANCAKES WITH VANILLA SAUCE

- *2 servings*

Ingredients

- Kaiserschmarrn
- 1 tbsp (willow) butter (or ghee)
- 3 egg
- 1 egg white
- 100 g cottage cheese ((granular cream cheese))
- 40 g organic cream cheese double cream stage
- 1 tablespoon of psyllium husk ground
- 1 TL Puderxucker
- Taste of rum
- Lemon juice
- Cinnamon
- Stevia
- Vanilla sauce
- 1 egg yolk
- 100 ml organic whipped cream at least 30% fat
- Vanilla

Preparation

Total time approx. 20min

Melt the butter or ghee in a pan over medium heat. Put the cottage cheese, cream cheese and eggs in a mixing bowl. Purée the whole, creating a smooth dough. Taste the dough with rum, cinnamon and stevia. Stir the psyllium husks into the dough. Separate AN egg and beat the egg white stiff. Then carefully lift it under the dough. Gently pour the dough into the hot pan. As soon as the bottom of the dough is lightly brown, quarter and turn the resulting pancake. Fry as long as necessary and turn several times, if necessary, until the Kaiserschmarrn has the desired color and consistency. Then chop the pieces to the desired size.

Vanilla sauce:

Put on a water bath, heat cream and vanilla in a water bath - do not cook. Add the egg yolk, stir the sauce well and serve it lightly cooled along with the Kaiserschmarrn.

(Macros - Calories 511, Carb. 3g, Protein 24g, Fat 42g)

LUNCH
PARSLEY ROOT AND CELERY CASSEROLE

- *4 servings*

Ingredients

- 350 g parsley root
- 350 g of celeriac
- 1 onion
- 1 tbsp coconut oil
- 200 ml organic whipped cream at least 30% fat
- 200 ml of milk
- 200 g Gouda (grated)
- 150 g bacon (diced)
- 1 toe garlic
- Salt
- Pepper
- Nutmeg

Preparation

Total time approx. 1hr 35min

Clean the vegetables, peel and cut into thin slices. Dice the onions and sauté in a large saucepan with 1 tablespoon of oil. Add the vegetables, add the cream and milk and simmer for about 10 minutes. Stir now and then. If not already done, grate the cheese and dice the bacon. Mix half of the cheese and the bacon under the vegetables, stir well. Press the garlic clove and add to the vegetables. Season the vegetables well with salt, pepper and nutmeg. Distribute everything in a casserole dish and bake at 200 ° C top / bottom heat (circulating air 180 ° C) for about 60 minutes.

(Macros - Calories 595, Carb. 12g, Protein 23g, Fat 47g)

DINNER
PUMPKIN SOUP
- *1 serving*

Ingredients
- Onion
- 1 toe garlic
- 1 butternut squash (about 500g)
- 400 ml of coconut milk
- 50 g Gouda (grated)
- Salt
- Pepper
- Ginger
- Chili
- 1 tbsp coconut oil

Preparation
Total time approx. 20min
Dice the onion and garlic and sauté in coconut oil in a pot. Wash the pumpkin and chop it into small pieces, add to the onions and cover with boiling water. Boil the pumpkin until it is completely soft and crushes. Add the coconut milk and season with the spices. Bring to a boil again briefly and then purée.
(Macros - Calories 282, Carb. 13g, Protein 5g, Fat 22g)

DAY   7

BREAKFAST
EGG CASSEROLE AVOCADO
- *2 serving*

Ingredients
- Aluminum foil
- 2 lawyers
- 4 big caliber eggs
- 1 pinch salt [optional]
- Pepper to taste [optional]
- 1 pinch Cayenne pepper
- 2 teaspoons fresh chive, finely chopped [optional]

Preparation
Total time approx. 20min

Preheat the oven to 220 ° C / 425 ° F. Cover with foil a baking sheet. Slice the avocados in half lengthwise and remove the core. Using a spoon, remove about a spoonful or more of avocado flesh to create a hollow large enough to deposit an egg. Put the avocados on the plate and fold the foil around the avocados to prevent them from tipping over. Alternatively put each lawyer in a ramekin. Break one egg into each avocado half taking care not to break the yolk. Add salt and pepper to taste. Add a pinch of Cayenne.

Place in the center of the oven and bake 15-18 min. Or until the whites have seared, and the yolks are still a little runny.

Garnish with chopped chives and serve.

Macros - calories 350, fat 29g, Net carb. 4g, protein 16g

LUNCH
AVOCADO BACON GRATIN
- *1 serving*

Ingredients
- 1 avocado (hate)
- 2 small tomatoes
- 50 g bacon
- 30 g (willow) butter
- 75 g Gouda

Preparation

Total time approx. 20min

Halve the avocado, remove the kernel, cut the pulp into small pieces. Dice the tomatoes and the bacon, put everything together with the butter in an ovenproof dish. Sprinkle the cheese over and bake everything at 180 ° C circulating air for about 15 minutes to the desired tan.

The recipe can be varied very easily. Instead of bacon, you can also use salami or another ham, like chicken breast strips or something.

Often you can also add peppers and a little more onion, depending on what the refrigerator just gives.

If you do not have an oven (work, for example), maybe you have a microwave with grill? It works very well too, so you just have to

see when the cheese runs dry and turns brown. Probably 5 minutes are enough. Tastes just as delicious.
(Macros - Calories 1063, Carb. 2g, Protein 28g, Fat 102g)

DINNER
KETOGENIC GNOCCHI IN GORGONZOLA SAUCE
- *3 servings*

Ingredients

- Gnocchi
- 400 g cream quark 40%
- 2 eggs
- 5 tablespoons guar gum
- 1 pinch of salt
- Herbs, spices (if you like)

- Sauce
- 200 g of Gorgonzola
- 200 ml organic whipped cream at least 30% fat
- Salt
- Pepper
- Parmesan

Preparation

Total time approx. 50mins

Making gnocchi dough: Put the quark, eggs and guar gum in a mixing bowl. It is best to stir the dough with a dough hook mixer. Please do not use a whisk, the dough will quickly become very tough. Let the dough rest for 15 minutes. Then he should be really tough, but no longer stick. If the dough is still sticky, add one tbsp guar gum extra, knead the dough well and let it rest for another 5 minutes. While swelling, you can already prepare the sauce.

Prepare the sauce:

Put the gorgonzola with the cream in a pan and let the cheese melt slowly over medium heat. Stir from time to time to make a nice creamy sauce. Season with salt, pepper and possibly some Parmesan to taste. Then set aside to keep warm.

Cook gnocchi and Fill a large pot with water, add some salt and let the water boil. Until the water boils, we finish the gnocchi. Put some guar gum on the worktop and place the dough out of the mixing bowl. Take a teaspoon, make it wet from time to time and use it to cut off the small amount of dough for gnocchi. Make a lot of little gnocchi balls out of it. If it sticks too much, simmer the dough with guar gum again. Take a fork and lightly press in the little balls so they have the typical gnocchi shape. Meanwhile, the water should boil. At this point, the table should already be ready, because now it is very fast. Put the finished gnocchi in the boiling water. When they swim on the water surface, they are done. If the water has not boiled again by then, it may be a short wait. Take the finished gnocchi and put it in the pan with the gorgonzola sauce. Panning once more in the sauce and then serve on a plate. Parmesan and fresh basil are enough.

(Macros - Calories 732, Carb. 4g, Protein 39g, Fat 61g)

WEEK 3

DAY 1

BREAKFAST
CAULIFLOWER BAKE
- *6 servings*

Ingredients
- 2 pieces of cauliflower (small)
- 300 g Gouda (grated)
- 250 g bacon (diced)
- 200 g organic whipped cream at least 30% fat
- 4 eggs
- Salt
- Pepper
- Nutmeg

Preparation
Total time approx. 45min

Bring a large pot of salted water to a boil. Divide the cauliflower into small florets and boil in salted water for about 10 minutes. Mix the eggs with the cream for at least 2 minutes, ideally 5 minutes. So, the egg cream is nice and creamy. Season with salt, pepper and nutmeg. Rub the cheese, dice the bacon, if it is not already diced, and mix everything with the egg cream. Because bite-fixed cauliflower in a casserole dish. Distribute the bacon and the egg cream-cheese-bacon mixture evenly on the cauliflower. Stir well again. Bake the casserole for about 25 minutes at 180 ° C convection (200 ° C top / bottom heat) until the cheese is golden brown.

(Macros - Calories 491, Carb. 5g, Protein 28g, Fat 36g)

LUNCH
VEGETABLE LASAGNA FROM THE SLOW COOKER
- *3 servings*

Ingredients
- 300 g minced meat
- 1 zucchini (small)
- 1 pepper
- 1 onion
- 1 toe garlic

- 150 g organic cream cheese double cream stage
- 150 g Gouda (grated)
- 400 g pizza tomatoes

Preparation

Total time approx. 3hrs 15mins

Dice the onions and sauté in coconut oil or butter in a pan, squeeze the garlic and add. Put minced meat in the pan and sauté well. Season with salt and pepper. Deglaze with the tomatoes and simmer until the liquid is largely overcooked. Peel the zucchini and cut into thin slices. Wash the peppers and cut into rings or strips. Now the lasagna is layered in the slow cooker: First lay out the bottom with zucchini strips, then layer some pepper rings, then add some ground beef and spread some cream cheese over the minced meat. Continue in this order. When finished, add the rest of the cream cheese and the grated cheese. Simmer the lasagna for 3-4 hours at high.

(Macros - Calories 582, Carb. 9g, Protein 35g, Fat 43g)

DINNER
BACON PIZZA

- *4 servings*

Ingredients

- 4 packs. Bacon, sliced
- 100 g bacon diced
- 1 stick of spring onion
- 3 tablespoons tomato paste
- 2 balls mozzarella
- 1 pepper
- 200 g of Gouda grated
- 100 g ham to taste, or salami
- 6-8 cocktail tomatoes

Preparation

Total time approx. 25mins

Lay out the bacon strips on a grill and braid as in the picture. Make sure that the discs are nicely close to each other so that it does not fall apart later. Possibly. also beat the corners and press something to have a nice edge. Now place the "Bacon-Pizza-

Floor" in the oven and grill until the top becomes slightly brown. Then take it out again, turn the bacon over with a large spatula and grate briefly again.

Bacon pizza ground:

Meanwhile, cut the onions into small pieces and sauté with the bacon cubes. Add the tomato puree and add a little water, so that the sauce is not liquid, but not too firm. Slice the mozzarella and cut the peppers into small cubes.

Once the pizza base has been grilled, take it out of the oven, you can switch off the grill. Carefully place the bacon tomato sauce on the pizza base, then place the mozzarella slices on top. If you do not have mozzarella, spread some ground Gouda on top. This way, the pizza topper keeps better. Now it's off to the pizza topping: Prove the pizza with the diced peppers, the tomato slices and the ham, just as you like it. Finally, spread the grated Gouda on the pizza. The entire pizza is now for about 10 minutes at 180 ° C top / bottom heat in the oven, or until the cheese has the desired tan.

(Macros - Calories 748, Carb. 6g, Protein 52g, Fat 57g)

DAY 2

BREAKFAST
QUICK AVOCADO TOAST

- *Servings: 2*

Ingredients

- 4 cloud breads
- 8 tablespoons of mayonnaise
- 4 large tomato slices
- 1 large avocado
- Salt and pepper (to your taste)

Preparation

Prepare the cloud bread the day before. Bake 4 rolls (you should get a golden color). Plug in the toaster and put the bread rolls in the toaster. Open and hollow the avocado. Cut them into quarters, then thin into slices. Put 2 tablespoons of mayonnaise,

a slice of tomato and a quarter of chopped avocado on each bun. Add salt and pepper to taste.
(Macros - Fat 52g, Protein 6g, Net carb. 3g, Calories 535)

LUNCH
BEEF STEW

- *Servings: 2*

Ingredients

- 450 g ground beef
- 1/2 green pepper
- 1/2 cup marinara sauce
- 1 tablespoon Dijon mustard
- 1 tablespoon soy sauce

Preparation

Total time approx. 20min

Chop green peppers and fry them with a little fat in the pan until tender. Do it on medium heat. Add ground beef, then divide it into small pieces using a wooden spoon or spatula. Hold the beef in the pan until the meat turns brown. Add marinara sauce, Dijon mustard and soy sauce. Season to taste with salt and pepper. Cook the whole thing until the beef is completely ready and the sauce slightly thickens.
(Macros - Fat 50g, Protein 38g, Net carb. 2g, Calories 640)

DINNER
SAFFRON CHICKEN

- *5 Serving*

Ingredients

- 6 Organic chicken thighs
- 2 tbsp olive oil
- 2.5 g saffron,
- 2 tbsp Curry Powder,
- 1 teaspoon cumin
- 1 teaspoon paprika powder
- Salt
- 2 tbsp of organic chicken broth

Preparation

Total time approx. 45min

Disassemble chicken thighs at the joint into two parts. To do this, cut the meat to the bone with a knife and then split the joint with a knife or poultry shears.

Heat olive oil in a large saucepan. Fry the chicken thighs. Season generously: Saffron, curry powder, cumin, paprika, salt and pure organic chicken broth drizzle over it. Turn the lid on and turn down the heat. The meat cooks in its own juice.

After 30 minutes, the meat is cooked. If you like, you can sear the individual parts in a pan in oil again. So, the chicken tastes even more intense and looks more beautiful.

(Macros - 416kcal, protein 37g, fat 27g, carbohydrates 5g)

DAY 3

BREAKFAST
BAKED CHORIZO

- *Servings: 2*

Ingredients

- 1/4 red pepper
- 1/4 green pepper
- 80 g chorizo sausage
- 1/2 cup grated mozzarella
- 4 large eggs

Preparation

Total time approx. 25min

Cut the red and green peppers into cubes and the chorizo into bite-sized pieces. Fry the chorizo sausage, transfer to a plate, then fry the paprika until soft. Gently grease 4 kills, pour in each pepper, chorizo and mozzarella. Add beaten egg to each ramekin, season with salt and pepper. Bake for 12 minutes at 180°C.

(Macros - Fat 32g, Protein 27g, Net carb 3g, Calories 418)

LUNCH
CHICKEN IN PARMESAN CHEESE

- *Servings: 2*

Ingredients

- 2 chicken breasts, 150-200 g each
- 1 large egg (beaten)
- 1/4 cup grated Parmesan cheese
- 55 grams of pork skins
- 1/2 cup marinara sauce

Preparation
Total time approx. 40min
With the help of a food processor, grind pork skins and Parmesan cheese until it has the consistency of breadcrumbs. Wrap the chicken breasts in the egg, and then in the low-carbohydrate coating that you just created. Cover the meat thoroughly. Bake coated chicken for 30 minutes. Use an oven heated to 190 ° C. About 5 minutes before removing the chicken from the oven, add marinara sauce to it. Serve the dish sprinkled with an additional portion of Parmesan cheese and dry spices of your choice.
(Macros - Fat 23g, Protein 52g, Net carb. 2g, Calories 425)

DINNER
SOUP VEGETABLES AND TEMPEH
- *2 serving*

Ingredients
- 2 cups vegetables soup
- 1 cup water 250 mL
- 1/3 cup unsweetened coconut milk
- 1/2 limes / limes, juice and zest
- 1 little Bok choy
- ½ dried red peppers, finely chopped
- 200 g shirataki noodles / konjac
- 4 teaspoons coconut oil
- 240 g tempeh, cut into cubes
- 1 teaspoon curry / curry powder
- 1 pinch salt [optional]
- Pepper to taste [optional]
- ½ carrots, finely grated
- ½ green onions / shallots, chopped
- 9 tablespoons bean sprouts

Preparation

Total time approx. 20min
Rinse the noodles with plenty of water to eliminate the odor and drain well. In a saucepan, bring broth, water, coconut milk, zest and lime juice to a boil. Add the Bok choy and red pepper. Reserve on a low heat. Meanwhile, heat a skillet over medium heat. Add noodles and cook for 2-3 minutes, stirring until all noodles are hot. Remove the noodles from the pan and set aside. In the skillet, heat the oil over medium-high heat. You need to jump cubes with tempeh curry. Jump until golden brown, about 5 min. Salt and pepper. Prepare the vegetables: Grate the carrots and finely slice the green onions. Spread in the bowls with the sprouts, noodles, tempeh cubes and cooking oil. Pour broth over. To serve.
(Macros - calories 480, Net carb.9g, protein 28g)

DAY 4

BREAKFAST
EGG AVOCADO WRAPPED IN BACON
- *2 servings*

Ingredients
- 330 g avocado
- 50 g egg
- 100 g bacon
- 20 g of coconut oil

Preparation

Total time approx. 25min

Cook the egg hard. Cut the avocado in half and carefully remove the core. Use a spoon to separate the flesh from the skin. If necessary, scrape out a bit more avocado from the core area, so that fits a boiled egg.

Place two strips of bacon horizontally and on top of a large board. Now place five more strips, beginning on the vertical strip of bacon, downwards. Fill the avocado with the egg and close the halves well. Put the stuffed avocado down on the bacon and roll up. Also wrap around with the length of bacon strips and press well. Heat the coconut oil in a pan and fry the avocado well on all sides. If the bacon coat is crispy all around, it can be served.
(Macros - Calories 516, Fat 47g, Carb. 15g, Protein 16g)

LUNCH
CRISPY BACON SALAD
2 Servings
Ingredients
- 130 g Bacon
- 2 teaspoons Salt
- 20 g Walnut halves
- 1 teaspoon Water
- 1 tbsp. spoons Stevia
- 40 g Blue cheese
- 1/4 pcs Pear
- 0.5 tsp Dijon mustard
- 0.5 tsp Whole Grain Mustard
- 2 tbsp. spoons Wine vinegar
- 2 teaspoons Olive oil
- 60 g Greenery

Preparation
Total time approx. 20min

Turn on the oven. Take a slice of bacon, sprinkle with 1 teaspoon of olive oil and salt on both sides. Fry in the oven until a golden-brown crisp appears for about 20-30 minutes. While you wait, chop the walnut into small pieces. Heat the pan over medium heat, add water and stevia to it, wait until it dissolves and add walnuts. Cook, stirring, for about 5 minutes, until the liquid thickens and caramelizes. Do not touch nuts until they have cooled. Dice the blue cheese, pear and set them aside. Make a green salad by adding mustard, wine vinegar, and olive oil. Remove the crispy bacon from the oven, let it cool, and then cut into cubes. Mix all the ingredients - the salad is ready.

(Macros - Calories 538, Fat 51.5g, Carb. 6.6g, Protein 12.7g)

DINNER
STUFFED CHICKEN BREASTS WITH MOZZARELLA
- *6 servings*

Ingredients
- 100 g Cream cheese
- 100 g Mozzarella Cheese Grated
- 300 g Frozen Spinach
- 3 pcs Chicken breast
- 1 tbsp. Olive oil
- 60 ml Tomato Sauce, Sugar Free
- 3 pcs Mozzarella cheese, slice (slice)
- Salt and pepper

Preparation
Total time approx. 40min
Put cream cheese, grated mozzarella and spinach in a bowl. Put in the microwave for a couple of minutes so that the cheese melts and you can mix everything to a cream. Make deep cross sections on chicken breasts, sprinkle with salt and pepper. Put the cheese mixture in the cuts. Put the chicken in a mold (use a cast-iron skillet) and put in an oven preheated to 180 ° C for 25 minutes. Then, switch the oven to grill mode and increase the temperature to 220 C. Lubricate the fillet with tomato sauce, put on each slice Mozzarella and bake for another 5 minutes.
(Macros - Calories 338, fat 18.3g, Carb.4.1g, Protein 37.9g)

DAY   5

BREAKFAST
A HEALTHY LEMON PIE WITHOUT SUGAR
- *Servings: 8*

Preparation
- 1/2 cup unsalted, melted butter
- 1¾ cup almond flour
- 1 cup powdered erythritol
- 3 medium lemons
- 3 large eggs

Preparation
Total time approx. 65min

Mix butter, 1 cup of almond flour, 1/4 cup of erythritol together and add a pinch of salt. Roll out evenly and transfer to a 20 × 20 cm sheet of parchment paper. Bake at 175 °C for 20 minutes. Then leave to cool for 10 minutes. In a bowl, grate one of the lemons, then squeeze all 3 lemons, add eggs, 3/4 cup erythritol, 3/4 cup almond flour and a pinch of salt. Mix the dough filling thoroughly. Pour the filling to the chilled bottom and bake for 25 minutes. Serve the cake decorated with lemon slices and powdered erythritol.
(Macros - Fat 26g, Protein 8g, Net carb 4g, Calories 272)

LUNCH
SALMON CUTLETS
- *2 Servings*

Ingredients
- 150 g Canned salmon
- 1 Egg
- 2 tbsp. Mayonnaise
- 1 Clove of garlic
- 1/4 teaspoon Ginger powder
- 2 tbsp. Olive oil
- Salt
- 1 Avocado (medium size)
- 80 ml Sour cream
- Cilantro
- 2 tbsp. Water
- 2 tbsp. Lemon juice

Preparation
Total time approx. 20min
Drain the salmon jar. In a bowl, combine fish, egg, mayonnaise, chopped garlic, ginger and salt. Blind 4 patties and fry over medium heat in olive oil for 4-5 minutes on each side (until light golden brown. For the sauce, mix the avocado pulp, sour cream, cilantro, a tablespoon of olive oil and lemon juice in a blender. Add water to obtain the desired consistency.
(Macros - Calories 566, fat 50g, Carb. 10g, Protein 19g)

DINNER
CARBONARA PASTA

- *4 servings*

Ingredients

- 20 g Butter
- 2 pcs Garlic (clove)
- 180 g Bacon
- 50 ml Dry white wine
- 4 g Egg
- 100 g Cream 33%
- 100 g Parmesan Cheese
- Ground pepper and salt

Preparation

Total time approx. 25min

Fry the garlic in butter, then add the sliced bacon. Fry for 2-3 minutes, then add the wine. Let the wine evaporate, then remove the pan from the heat, transfer the bacon to paper so that it cools and becomes crispy. Remove the pan from the heat, transfer the bacon to the paper so that it cools and becomes crispy. In a bowl, mix the yolks, cream and Parmesan until smooth. Boil shirataki. Put the pasta, bacon in a cold frying pan, pour the creamy mixture, salt and put on medium heat. Stir the paste until the mixture thickens. It is important not to overcook Carbonara so that the yolks do not burn. Put the pasta in plates and sprinkle with freshly ground pepper.

(Macros - Calories 461, fat 40.5g, Carb. 3.5g, Protein 23.7g)

DAY 6

BREAKFAST
CHIA COFFEE PUDDING

- *1 serving*

Ingredients

- 4 tbsp. Chia seeds
- 150 ml Iced coffee
- 150 ml Coconut milk
- 1 tbsp. Almond oil
- 1 tbsp. Erythritol
- Cinnamon
- Salt

Preparation

Total time approx. 5min

Put all the ingredients in a bowl and mix thoroughly. Cover and refrigerate overnight.

(Macros - Calories 282, Fat 24g, Carb. 12.6g, Protein 5.9g)

LUNCH
CREAM BROCCOLI SOUP WITH CHEESE

- *4 servings*

Ingredients

- 2 cups Frozen Broccoli
- 1 Medium Carrot
- 1 Small onion
- 2 tbsp. Olive oil
- 1 teaspoon Garlic powder
- Salt and pepper
- 2 cups Chicken bouillon
- 50 g Fresh spinach
- 1/2 cup Cream
- 100 g Cheddar Cheese
- 100 g Gouda Cheese

Preparation

Total time approx. 25

Heat the olive oil in a saucepan (deep frying pan) over medium heat. Fry onions and carrots for 1-2 minutes, then add broccoli, garlic, salt and pepper. Fry for another minute, stirring constantly. Pour in the broth, mix and simmer for 8-10 minutes until the vegetables are soft. Turn off the heat, add the cream and mix. Pour half the soup into a blender and add half the spinach.

Grind to the desired consistency. Then, repeat the process with the second half. Pour the mashed soup back into the pan (deep pan), add the cheese and stir until it is completely melted.
(Macros - Calories 277, Fat 21g, Carb. 4g, Protein 15g)

DINNER
CHICKEN SALAD
- *4servings*

Ingredients
- 450 g Boneless chicken thighs
- 30 g Butter
- 225 g Bacon
- 110 g Cherry tomatoes
- 275 g Lettuce or Romaine Salad
- Salt and pepper
- 175 ml Mayonnaise
- ½ teaspoon Garlic powder

Preparation
Total time approx. 30min

Fry the bacon in butter until golden brown and remove from the pan. Put chopped chicken thigh fillet in the same skillet, salt and pepper. Sauté until cooked. Put lettuce, tomatoes in a bowl, put chicken and bacon on top. Combine the mayonnaise with garlic powder and season the salad.
(Macros - Calories 837, fat 78g, Carb.4g, Protein 28g)

DAY 7

BREAKFAST
OMELET WITH MUSHROOMS
- *1 serving*

Ingredients
- 3 Eggs
- 100 g Mushrooms
- 30 g Butter
- 30 g Parmesan Cheese
- 30 g Onion
- Salt and pepper

Preparation
Total time approx. 15min

Put 20 g of oil in a skillet and turn on medium heat. Once the butter has melted, put the chopped onion and fry for 2-3 minutes until it begins to darken. Then, add the mushrooms and sauté until tender. If you take pre-boiled chanterelles or small mushrooms, then frying will take no more than five minutes.
Remove the finished mixture from the pan. Beat the eggs in a bowl, add salt, pepper and beat with a whisk until smooth. Put the remaining 10 g of butter in a skillet, allow to melt and pour the future omelet as soon as the omelet grabs from the bottom, and the top is still liquid, sprinkle it with grated Parmesan and put mushrooms with onions on one half. Gently pry the omelet on one side with a spatula and fold it like a book. Turn off the fire, cover and let the omelet stand for five minutes, until it reaches readiness
(Macros - Calories 510, Fat 43g, Carb. 4g, Protein 25g)

<u>LUNCH</u>
DELICATE SALAD WITH CHICKEN AND AVOCADO
- *4 servings*

Ingredients
- 150 g Ready Chicken Fillet
- 2 Avocado
- 6 pcs Hard Boiled Egg
- 8 pcs Bacon slice
- 2 tbsp. Greek yogurt or heavy cream
- 2 tbsp. Mayonnaise
- 2 teaspoons Lemon juice
- 20 g Fresh cilantro chopped
- Salt and pepper

Preparation
Total time approx. 20min
Dice the chicken, avocado and eggs, put them in a bowl, add yogurt, mayonnaise, lemon juice and cilantro. Salt, pepper to taste and mix thoroughly. Fry the bacon until crispy. Break it into small pieces and sprinkle salad.
(Macros - Calories 386, Fat 30g, Carb. 8g, Protein 23g)

DINNER
HOMEMADE KETO DUMPLINGS
- *20 servings*

Ingredients
- 96 g Almond flour
- 24 g Coconut Flour
- 2 teaspoons Xanthan gum
- Salt
- 2 teaspoons Apple vinegar
- 1 pc Egg
- 3-5 teaspoons Water
- 400 g Spinach
- 250 g Ricotta cheese
- 40 g Parmesan Cheese
- 30 g Roasted pine nuts
- 1/4 teaspoon Nutmeg
- 1 pc Yolk
- Butter for frying
- Garlic, Parmesan, Thyme, Cherry Tomatoes

Preparation

Total time approx. 45mins

Combine almond, coconut flour, gum and salt in a food processor in pulse mode. Add apple cider vinegar, then beat the egg. Stir and add water over a teaspoon until the dough forms into a ball. The dough should be tight. Wrap the dough in a film and remember it for a couple of minutes. Leave the dough for 15 minutes at room temperature, and then refrigerate for 45 minutes. Heat olive oil in a pan over medium heat. Slightly fry the garlic, add the spinach and fry until softened. Put on a board and chop. Combine spinach with ricotta, Parmesan cheese, fried pine nuts, nutmeg, salt and egg yolk. Divide the dough into two parts and roll each between two layers of parchment. Lay out a tablespoon of the filling, cover with a second layer and press the dough with your fingers between the filling. Cut out future ravioli, transfer them to a baking sheet and freeze for 15 minutes. Heat butter in a pan, add slices of garlic and thyme. When the garlic begins to brown, add chilled ravioli. Sauté them until golden, one or two minutes on each side. Sprinkle the prepared ravioli with Parmesan and garnish with cherry tomatoes.

(Macros - Calories 88, Fat 6g, Carb. 3g, Protein 4g)

www.ingramcontent.com/pod-product-compliance
Ingram Content Group UK Ltd.
Pitfield, Milton Keynes, MK11 3LW, UK
UKHW022225230426
12048UKWH00016BA/1063